Managing Global Health Security

Managing Global Health Security

The World Health Organization and Disease Outbreak Control

Adam Kamradt-Scott
Senior Lecturer, University of Sydney, Australia

palgrave
macmillan

First published 2015 by
PALGRAVE MACMILLAN

Palgrave Macmillan in the UK is an imprint of Macmillan Publishers Limited, registered in England, company number 785998, of Houndmills, Basingstoke, Hampshire RG21 6XS.

Palgrave Macmillan in the US is a division of St Martin's Press LLC, 175 Fifth Avenue, New York, NY 10010.

Palgrave is the global academic imprint of the above companies and has companies and representatives throughout the world.

Palgrave® and Macmillan® are registered trademarks in the United States, the United Kingdom, Europe and other countries.

ISBN: 978–0–230–36931–3

This book is printed on paper suitable for recycling and made from fully managed and sustained forest sources. Logging, pulping and manufacturing processes are expected to conform to the environmental regulations of the country of origin.

A catalogue record for this book is available from the British Library.

Library of Congress Cataloging-in-Publication Data

Kamradt-Scott, Adam, 1974–, author.
    Managing global health security: the World Health Organization and disease outbreak control / Adam Kamradt-Scott.
        p. ; cm.
    Includes bibliographical references.
    ISBN 978–0–230–36931–3
    I. Title.
    [DNLM: 1. World Health Organization.   2. Communicable Disease Control—legislation & jurisprudence.   3. Disease Outbreaks—prevention & control.   4. Global Health.   5. Health Policy.   6. Health Services Administration.   7. International Cooperation.   WA 33.1]
    RA441
    362.1—dc23   2015001022

2|22|19

To all those quiet achievers who have striven to make the world a healthier and safer place through your dedicated and unyielding public service. While often unsung, you are heroes nonetheless.

Contents

List of Table   viii

Acknowledgements   ix

List of Acronyms   x

Introduction   1

1 The Legal Basis for the WHO's Global Health Security
   Mandate and Authority   21

2 The WHO's Classical Approach to Disease Eradication   45

3 Securitization and SARS: A New Framing?   79

4 New Powers for a New Age? Revising and Updating the IHR   101

5 Pandemic Influenza: 'The Most Feared Security Threat'   125

6 Global Health Security and Its Discontents   151

Concluding Remarks   181

Notes   191

Bibliography   195

Index   223

List of Table

6.1   WHO work programme priorities   161

Acknowledgements

Inevitably, as with any project that has literally taken over a decade to be realized, there are many people to thank. My academic colleagues have, in various ways, supported me through the years in guiding, advising, and, at times, politely disagreeing with and correcting my ideas and observations. Indeed, I have been fortunate throughout my career to rub shoulders with a veritable 'who's who' of experts in global health governance, including Sara Davies, Stefan Elbe, Christian Enemark, Harley Feldbaum, Sophie Harman, Kelley Lee, Colin McInnes, Anne Roemer-Mahler, Simon Rushton, Frank Smith III, Owain Williams, and Jeremy Youde, just to name a few. Special thanks also go to Sarah Phillips and Lucy Fiske, who while not researching global health per se have served to inspire and challenge my preconceptions of what academics can do, and to my colleagues at the Marie Bashir Institute for Infectious Diseases and Biosecurity, especially Grant Hill-Cawthorne, Ben Marais, Siobhan Mor, and Tania Sorrell. Collectively and individually you have all encouraged and inspired me along this journey, and I have tremendously benefited not only from your insights and expertise but also your friendship. Thank you.

I am most grateful to Sandy Cocksedge, Fernando Gonzalez-Martin, David Heymann, Anne Marie Huvos, Bill Kean, Anne Kerr-Godal, David Nabarro, Isabelle Nuttall, and Guénaël Rodier, who over emails, cups of coffee and the occasional glass of wine helped clarify the inner workings of the WHO. Thank you for your anecdotes, insights, and stories; I only hope that I have done some justice to the extraordinarily valuable work to which you have dedicated your lives.

Sincere thanks also to the anonymous and not-so-anonymous reviewers, whose comments helped improve the quality of the book. Of course, any remaining faults and errors are entirely my own. Heartfelt thanks also are due to the editorial team at Palgrave for their long-suffering patience. Thank you.

Lastly, I thank my family, especially my mother and sister, who supported me when I had this crazy idea of changing career paths. I cannot possibly articulate in words what you mean to me, nor how much your love and support have helped make this possible.

List of Acronyms

AFRO	African Regional Office of the World Health Organization
ASEAN	Association of South East Asian Nations
BCG	Bacille Calmette-Guérin
CBRN	Chemical, Biological, Radiological and Nuclear
CDC	Centres for Disease Control and Prevention
CSR	Communicable Disease Surveillance and Response Unit
DDT	Dichloro-Diphenyl-Trichloroethane
DOTS	Directly Observed Treatment, Short-course
EB	Executive Board
EU	European Union
EMC	Emerging and Other Communicable Diseases
EMRO	Eastern Mediterranean Regional Office
EVD	Ebola Virus Disease
FAO	Food and Agriculture Organization
GDEP	Global DOTS Expansion Plan
GDF	Global TB Drug Facility
GIS	Geographical Information System
GISN	Global Influenza Surveillance Network
GISRS	Global Influenza Surveillance and Response System
GOARN	Global Outbreak Alert and Response Network
GPEI	Global Polio Eradication Initiative
GPHIN	Global Public Health Information Network
HCW	Healthcare workers
HIV	Human Immunodeficiency Virus
IAEA	International Atomic Energy Agency
ICAO	International Civil Aviation Organization
IGM	Inter-Governmental Meeting
IGWG	Inter-Governmental Working Group
IHR	International Health Regulations
IO	International Organization
ISEP	Intensified Smallpox Eradication Programme
ISR	International Sanitary Regulations
LNHO	League of Nations Health Organization
MDGs	Millennium Development Goals
MDRTB	Multi-Drug Resistant Tuberculosis
MEP	Malaria Eradication Programme

MSF	Médecins Sans Frontières
NFP	National Focal Point
NGO	Non-Government Organization
NIC	National Influenza Centre
ODA	Official Development Assistance
OIE	Office International des Epizooties (World Organization for Animal Health)
OIHP	Office Internationale d'Hygiene Publique
PAHO	Pan American Health Organization
PASB	Pan American Sanitary Bureau
PASO	Pan American Sanitary Organization
PHEIC	Public Health Emergency of International Concern
PIP	Pandemic Influenza Preparedness
SARS	Severe Acute Respiratory Syndrome
SEP	Smallpox Eradication Programme
TB	Tuberculosis
UN	United Nations
US	United States
UNAIDS	Joint United Nations Programme for HIV/AIDS
UNDP	United Nations Development Programme
UNESCO	United Nations Educational, Scientific and Cultural Organization
UNICEF	United Nations Children's Fund
UNMEER	United Nations Mission for Ebola Emergency Response
UNRRA	United Nations Relief and Rehabilitation Administration
UNSIC	United Nations System Influenza Coordinator
USSR	Union of Soviet Socialist Republics
WHA	World Health Assembly
WHO	World Health Organization
WIC	World Influenza Centre
WTO	World Trade Organization
WWI	World War I
WWII	World War II

Introduction

In the early hours of 15 March 2003, Dr Hoe Nam Leong was returning to Singapore from New York with his pregnant wife and mother-in-law on Singapore Airlines flight SQ25. The doctor had only arrived in the United States a few days earlier to attend a medical conference, but within a day of arrival he had started to feel unwell. On visiting a hospital in New York Dr Leong was diagnosed with pneumonia, and so, gathering his family, he decided to return to Singapore early to start treatment. The doctor did not suspect at the time that he may have contracted the same unidentified respiratory illness that he had been treating a patient in Singapore for, but before boarding the plane Dr Leong contacted a colleague to inform him that he was feeling unwell and would be flying home. Demonstrating his professional commitment to the well-being of others, whilst on the aircraft Dr Leong isolated himself at the back of the plane – so as to avoid potentially infecting other passengers – and settled in for the long flight. On its scheduled stopover in Frankfurt, Germany, however, Dr Leong, his family, and the rest of the passengers were confronted by a scene straight out of a Hollywood blockbuster when a contingent of medical doctors dressed in biological isolation suits boarded the plane and escorted the doctor and his family off the plane and directly to hospital. Dr Leong was not to know at the time that his phone call to a colleague in Singapore where he had revealed he was feeling unwell and was boarding a plane had prompted an international crisis of the highest order. Indeed, in response to the doctor's decision to fly home, health authorities in Singapore, the United Kingdom, and Germany coordinated their efforts with the World Health Organization (WHO) in Geneva, Switzerland, to locate the doctor and his family and isolate them in order to prevent the spread of a novel, unknown disease. Fortunately, the doctor, his family, and a 22-year-old female flight attendant who also became infected eventually made a full recovery, and the disease was not transmitted to any of the other passengers on the plane or to the delegates at the medical conference he attended. Worldwide, however, the novel disease that subsequently became known as Severe Acute Respiratory Syndrome (SARS) infected over 8,500 people – and caused the death of over 916 – before it was eventually contained in July 2003.

For many, the 2003 SARS outbreak proved a timely 'wake-up call' regarding the nature of contemporary disease events. By the beginning of the 21st century humanity had achieved a level of spatial, temporal, and cognitive interconnectedness that had never before been witnessed. This phenomenon, commonly described as 'globalization', has irrevocably changed how we experience our world and interact with each other (Lee 2003). At the corporeal level, people and livestock can now traverse the entire planet within 24 hours, aided by technological advances in transport. At the same time, due to human ingenuity in telecommunications, we can now be made aware of events occurring on the other side of the planet within mere seconds. This brave new world of global interconnectedness has brought with it both challenges and benefits, but perhaps none more so than in the pathogenic environment. For along with the advances in science and technology that have generated remarkable medical advances to cure illness and disease, microbes – and the diseases they cause – can now also move readily around the world at unprecedented speed to reach geographical locations previously unrealized.

The WHO has a central role to play in the international prevention, control, and eradication of infectious diseases. It is a responsibility that was ascribed to the first truly universal intergovernmental health agency in 1948 when the organization was founded, and is listed amongst 22 functions or duties that the organization is expected to fulfil. Throughout its more than 60 years of operation, the WHO has consistently sought to execute its responsibilities in this area by assisting governments to prevent, control, and ideally eradicate disease, albeit to varying degrees of success. The majority of this activity has occurred under the organization's explicit public health mandate to serve as the 'directing and coordinating authority in international health' (WHO 2005a, p. 2 – see Article 2(a) of the WHO Constitution). In 2001, however, the WHO's member states passed a resolution that described the organization's efforts to better manage naturally occurring infectious disease outbreaks and epidemics, as well as the risks posed by biological agents, as 'global health security' (WHO 2001a). A few years later, this concept was further expanded upon in the 2007 World Health Report that described global public health security as 'the activities required, both proactive and reactive, to minimize vulnerability to acute public health events that endanger the collective health of populations living across geographical regions and international boundaries' (WHO 2007a, p. ix).

Global health security has subsequently been adopted as a core theme of the WHO's agenda, and has been used as a conceptual device to reorder the organization's programmes and activities. Moreover, health security has become a didactic tool that government officials, health professionals, and academics the world over have utilized to argue for anything from increased healthcare spending, capacity building, and health system strengthening, to the passage of new laws and regulations designed to enhance surveillance, curtail civil liberties, regulate behaviour, or facilitate technical cooperation at the national, regional, and international levels. It has given rise to new intergovernmental forums such as the Global Health Security Initiative and the European Commission's Health Security Committee, the passage of numerous bilateral and several multilateral agreements such as the revised International Health Regulations (2005) and the 2011 Pandemic Influenza Preparedness (PIP) Framework, and has prompted the allocation of billions of dollars to enhance governments' capabilities to respond to public health emergencies via initiatives such as the Global Health Security Agenda. Health security has, in short, become a rallying cry for a host of actors to reorder contemporary political, economic, and social life.

As the popularity of the concept has continued to grow, so too has the scope of issues that purportedly fall under its purview. Whereas throughout the majority of the previous century the connections between health and security were only seen to be associated with the risk of biological warfare (Fidler and Gostin 2008), recognition of the links between these two concepts has since expanded to include bioterrorism, disease outbreaks (irrespective of whether they are naturally occurring or intentionally orchestrated), human security, as well as the risks presented by dual-use technologies and emerging life sciences research (McInnes 2015). Accompanying this expansion of topics has also been the recognition of the wider societal impacts that such events can generate, particularly in terms of potential disruption to critical infrastructure and services, law and order issues, as well as more diverse impacts on social, economic, and military functioning. This recognition has in turn led to calls for greater involvement by actors not traditionally associated with the health sector to participate in planning and preparation activities. In the context of the WHO as the directing and coordinating authority in international health, the organization has witnessed its portfolio of responsibilities grow and multiply, and as will be explored in greater depth later, the WHO subsequently sought – and importantly, successfully obtained – several new powers that are intended to help the organization respond more rapidly and effectively to public health emergencies of international significance.

The WHO's comparatively recent adoption and deployment of language describing pathogens as 'threats' signifies a deeper change in the organization's approach to managing disease-related events. Admittedly the description of infectious diseases as threats to international security did not commence with the WHO; rather, it began in the early 1990s with various prominent individuals and institutions emphasizing the hazard that emerging and re-emerging infectious diseases presented (see Fidler 1996, Hughes 1998, Smith III 2014). The WHO's decision in 2001 to actively engage with and promote this worldview has, however, marked a distinct shift in the way in which the organization traditionally approaches disease outbreaks. Indeed, it signalled a move away from viewing such occurrences as natural events that should be handled exclusively by medical professionals to a recognition that disease outbreaks may not always be innocent, that the consequences arising from such events can have profound social, economic, and political impacts, and that mitigating their spread and effects often requires more than just the involvement of trained public health experts. This recognition has in turn prompted the WHO to strengthen its disease outbreak policies and procedures while also seeking several new powers to better coordinate the containment and elimination of disease. Exploring this evolution in the WHO's approach to managing global health security is the motivation behind this book.

Yet while many within the international community have embraced the WHO's move towards viewing health issues in security terms, it has also had its detractors. In this, the criticisms from the organization's member states have broadly followed two key trajectories and both sets of concerns have, at their core, the suggestion that the WHO has engaged in an unacceptable form of 'mission creep', which is when international organizations (IOs) seek to extend their powers or mandate beyond their original delegated purpose and function (Stone 2008). The first set of concerns has its basis in the continuing contestation surrounding the role, authority, and autonomy of IOs within contemporary international relations. When confronted with proposals to extend the WHO's investigative powers to enhance global health security, for example, a number of countries from the Middle East, Latin America, and Asia argued that such moves would fundamentally alter the organization's role and purpose from that of a public health agency to a security institution (Fidler 2005, Kamradt-Scott et al. 2012, Weir 2015). Governments have also been observed to question whether the WHO has obtained a sufficient mandate from its member states to describe its work in security terms (Tayob 2008).

A second and related set of concerns pertains to the concept of health security itself. Here, a small proportion of the WHO's member states that to date has included such countries as Brazil, Thailand, Indonesia, and India have expressed reservations about the organization's adoption of security-related concepts and language in discussing public health issues. The basis upon which these concerns have been raised relates to the lack of conceptual clarity over what the term 'health security' means and the scope of issues that it apparently applies to. These countries have asserted that, given their own objections, there is evidently no consensus on the WHO's use of this term, and accordingly the organization should refrain from using such language until further discussions are held (Aldis 2008, Tayob 2008).

As some might additionally expect, the discontent evidenced in the policy world has also been replicated in academe and followed multiple trajectories. Maclean (2008) has observed, for example, that the critiques may be conceived as falling into two distinct, albeit related, categories. The first 'involves a normative concern' with the effect on health outcomes that can arise from too closely associating health and security (ibid., p. 476). This line of reasoning maintains that while many additional financial and material resources can often be gained by highlighting the 'threat' nature of diseases, it can also necessitate the involvement of military institutions or other actors that hold divergent views on how the threat should be managed – perspectives that are inconsistent with traditional public health objectives. As several authors have gone on to note, these actors and the views they hold can have a number of unintended consequences. Elbe (2006), for example, has highlighted the risks associated with the securitization of infectious diseases when people carrying the Human Immunodeficiency Virus (HIV) are described as a threat to national security instead of the virus, while Selgelid and Enemark (2008) have underlined the danger of ethical and human rights infringements when security and disease are too closely aligned. Likewise, other authors such as Rushton (2011) and Stevenson and Moran (2015) have argued that the merging of health and security has resulted in some diseases being prioritized over other more pressing health needs because of the 'threat' they present to Western, high-income country interests. Correspondingly, the normative implication arising from these critiques is that the securitization of health is effectively morally compromised, and by default, the WHO's participation in this agenda is inappropriate, as it either tempers public health priorities or overlooks the needs of the most vulnerable.

As Maclean (2008) additionally notes, the second area of discontent to emerge over the conjoining of health and security has been from within the field of security studies and some of its practitioners. This line of argumentation reflects a general dissatisfaction with the broadening of security studies to include 'human security', as opposed to a specific objection to the annexation of health per se. As conceived in the 1994 United Nations Development Report, human security argues to replace the state as the referent object of security with humans (UNDP 1994). In so doing, it enables a re-categorization of what constitutes legitimate 'threats' with issues such as disease, unemployment, environmental hazards, hunger, and the like, gaining priority over more traditional threats such as military incursions and armed conflict. Various writers such as Paris (2001) and Macfarlane (2004) have argued that linking non-traditional issues such as health with security further diminishes the conceptual and political utility of security. Others have argued that the promise of human security is inherently flawed, serving to further entrench existing power imbalances that do nothing to help the poor and vulnerable (McCormack 2008). Yet despite all of the protestations regarding the practical or conceptual utility of the human security agenda, there has been broad acceptance that issues such as health do have a legitimate bearing on security, irrespective of whether one takes a state-centric or individually focused approach.

Why this book?

Aside from the billions of dollars that have been allocated and spent purportedly on enhancing 'global health security' or the extent to which health issues have come to feature on foreign policy agendas of late, why is a volume of this nature important? Said another way, why bother reading this book? Ultimately, this book has three key, interrelated objectives. The first is to highlight the significance of IOs, and specifically the WHO, to contemporary political life.

The role, authority, and autonomy of IOs continue to remain fiercely contested issues in contemporary international relations. Often accused of various misnomers such as their 'democratic deficit', their apparent incapacitating 'politicization', their dysfunctional behaviour, and for their perceived failures and/or inaction (Beigbeder 1987, Dutt 1995, Nye 2001, Barnett and Finnemore 2004), IOs are regularly condemned by governments, policy-makers, activists, and academics alike. They are, in short, habitually accused of not performing as intended. Given this rather persistent state of affairs, it is often difficult to assess whether such criticisms are in fact justified, and whether IOs are truly the self-aggrandizing, self-seeking tyrants that some suggest they are (Barnett and Finnemore 1999), or whether it is more a case that IOs are simply misrepresented, innocuous entities, merely trying to fulfil their mission in a world of competing agendas, interests, and priorities.

While the truth may be somewhere in between, the debate regarding the utility and benefit of delegating to IOs is not, by any means, a new phenomenon. Indeed, the study of IOs has a long pedigree within the discipline of International Relations (IR), for many years existing as the dominant focus of the discipline since its inception in 1919. Over the years, investigations surrounding these entities have ranged from scrutinizing how various post-war institutions addressed the problems they were created to resolve, to the study of power and how it was being exercised, and the influence of norms, rules, and principles in the form of 'international regimes' (Martin and Simmons 1998). As critics have occasionally noted, however, these analyses have rarely generated policy-relevant insights, with the result that IOs have been relegated to a minor field of inquiry (Rochester 1986). In this, aside from a few recent works (see Lee 2009, Chorev 2012), the WHO occupies an even smaller sphere of investigation. This is despite the fact that the WHO has been, and continues to be, often highly regarded by policy-makers and health practitioners alike as the most efficient and effective IO of all of the specialized agencies of the UN system (see, for example, Peabody 1995). This book seeks to address this imbalance and underline the importance of this particular IO to addressing the needs of the world's poorest and most vulnerable.

The second and related objective is to evaluate the role the WHO plays in preventing, controlling, and ideally eliminating, infectious diseases. As noted above, this function is currently listed in the WHO Constitution as one amongst 22 duties that the organization is expected to fulfil. Yet, while it may be tempting to ascribe the mitigation of infectious diseases the same value as these other duties, as this book will seek to evidence, the eradication of epidemics and pandemics exists as the WHO's chief function and the primary reason behind the organization's creation.

In fact, the position this book adopts is that the control and eradication of infectious diseases, security and the WHO have been intimately connected since the organization's founding. At the time when the IO's constitutive treaty was being negotiated in 1946, the focus was on using health as an apolitical vehicle for ensuring peace – health was a means to achieving security, or health-for-security. Over time, however, and by the arrival of the new millennium, worldviews had perceptibly shifted, with the outcome being that health was increasingly viewed as a legitimate security objective in itself – health has become synonymous with security, or health-as-security. Associated with this change – which has come about as a result of the technological advances in transport, population increases, environmental change, intensification of agricultural practices, and altered land pattern use – has been the recognition that epidemics and pandemics will likely prove to be a regular feature of human existence for many years to come. In view of that reality, as the directing and coordinating authority in international health matters the WHO will continue to play a large role in managing such events, and it is thereby wise to understand the limitations and constraints that the organization confronts.

Having said this, this book does not seek to provide an apologist account of the WHO. Nor does it seek to absolve the organization of its culpabilities and past mistakes, or even argue that the IO be granted additional powers to fulfil its mandate of eradicating infectious disease. The WHO, like any major institution and bureaucracy, has numerous faults, flaws, and inefficiencies – several of which this volume will highlight and discuss. Instead, the focus of this work is to evaluate the WHO's approach to controlling and eradicating infectious diseases (now understood as 'global health security'), paying particular attention to how the organization's management of this important public policy area has evolved and adapted over time.

In so doing, the book sets out to achieve its third objective of highlighting the role that ideas, arguments, and belief structures – and the individuals that hold them – have played in shaping the evolution of global health policy towards disease eradication. Indeed, in one sense the turn towards viewing infectious diseases as security threats can be viewed as just the latest development in a long line of ideas influencing and shaping the WHO's approach to global public health. As other works have explored, various ideas and belief structures such as human rights or economics have periodically come to prominence to inform public health policy and practice at the national level (see, for example, Smith 2013a, Smith III 2014). Moreover, these same ideas – or variants along the same themes – have often demonstrated a notable and profound impact upon not only the WHO as an institution (for example, see Chorev 2012), but also global health governance (GHG) practices more generally (Ollila 2005, Shiffman 2009, Davies 2010, Harman 2012, McInnes et al. 2012, 2014, Youde 2012). As such, the following analysis does not seek to simply recount a history of the WHO per se, nor track the ebb and flow of ideas in public health. Rather, the focus of this particular work is to place the evolution of the WHO's approach to managing global health security within its historical and political context, noting – where relevant – the influence and impact certain ideas have provoked along the way. Said another way, it is difficult to appreciate the evolution of the WHO's overall approach to controlling and eliminating infectious diseases without also understanding the impact of certain ideas within their historical context.

Theories, distinctions, and definitions

As may already be discernable, the following analysis adopts a constructivist approach to analysing the WHO and its management of global health security. Having said this, there are also two major theoretical frameworks that underpin the following work. The first of these is what has been described as Principal-Agent (PA) theory. Emanating from the field of economics, PA theory's focus on institutions, information asymmetries, and the processes of delegation has prompted widespread interest amongst political scientists hoping to explain 'real-world problems' (Elgie 2002, p. 187). The basic premise of PA theory is that a particular type of relationship develops when 'one party, the *principal*, enters into a contractual agreement with a second party, the *agent*, and delegates to the latter responsibility for carrying out a function or set of tasks on the principal's behalf' (Kassim and Menon 2003, p. 122, italics original). The relationship described between the principal and agent thereby corresponds well with the relationship that conventionally exists between IOs and their contracting parties (i.e. member states), and PA theory has subsequently become the dominant theoretical framework applied in contemporary IO studies (see, for example, Elsig 2010, Chorev 2012, Green and Colgan 2012, Oestreich 2012).

One of the more interesting facets of PA theory, however, is that it is assumed that agents can often develop divergent interests or preferences from their principals, and then act on those interests. This phenomenon has been described as *agency slack*, and it is generally held that there are two types of slack: *shirking*, where agents intentionally avoid executing their delegated functions or duties, and *slippage*, where agents slip the constraints of their principals to exercise their own preferences

(Hawkins et al. 2006). The ability of IOs to engage in agency slack though is also highly dependent upon two additional factors: the institutional design of the IO and how much autonomy the organization is capable of effecting. More specifically, the level of autonomy that an IO is capable of exercising (to be able to either shirk or slip its delegation contract) is contingent upon the control mechanisms member states have built into the IO's structure or institutional design. The constraints that member states (principals) commonly use to retain oversight of IOs and prevent transaction costs from arising normally tend to be of an economic or legal nature, prohibiting the organization from committing resources to certain specific areas or defining, through legislation, the areas considered to be within the competence of one or more IOs. Alternatively, they may be of a more technical or political nature, preventing the IO from commenting on certain issues or influencing the number and/or make-up of staff employed. Essentially, member states may choose a variety of means – or mechanisms of control – to prevent agency slack or mission creep occurring; it is in this regard that *IO autonomy* has been defined as 'the range of potential independent action available to an agent after the principal has established mechanisms of control' (ibid., p. 8). IO autonomy can therefore be differentiated from autonomy that is more generally equated with the ability to self-govern or freedom from external control.

Like many IOs, the WHO's relationship with its principals (member states) is a complicated one. In their work, Lyne et al. (2006) distinguish between two discrete models of complex principal relationships, noting that the most common type within international relations is that of a 'collective principal', which is when multiple actors enjoy authority over a common delegation contract for an agent. The inherent problem with this type of relationship, however, is that where principals' (member states) preferences diverge (otherwise described as 'preference heterogeneity' – see Hawkins et al. 2006) it can create political space for agency slack to emerge. Furthermore, principals experiencing preference heterogeneity are less likely to delegate to an agent in the first instance or to amend an existing delegation contract (ibid., pp. 20–1). As Weaver (2007, p. 496) has gone on to observe though, agency slack may not always be the fault of the agent, especially when 'one or more principals thwart the efforts of other principals to employ control mechanisms to monitor or direct agent behaviour'. This, therefore, speaks to the rather complicated nature of IO principal-agent relationships whenever there are multiple independent (sovereign) actors delegating to one agent.

On the converse side, it must also be appreciated that the agent – in this case, the WHO – is not necessarily a homogenous entity, nor can it always be assumed to exhibit preference homogeneity.[1] IOs are instead intrinsically complex entities, comprised of multiple departments, divisions, and sections, that can hold a variety of divergent, even contradictory views, cultures, and opinions as easily as the societies of the principals they serve. Moreover, subdivisions of an IO tasked with specific responsibilities of high political importance (such as coordinating international responses to disease outbreaks) may be more sensitive to and/or perceive themselves to be more answerable to member states' concerns than the larger bureaucracy, which in turn can contribute to internal preference heterogeneity. For these reasons, the WHO is best considered as a *collective agent*, which is 'an agent made up of more than one bureaucratic actor that is subject to a single contract with its principal' (Graham 2014, p. 369).

Furthermore, in the specific context of the WHO, the organization appears to have engendered a somewhat unique IO pathology in consigning its principals into different categories of importance as they relate to the organization's global health security mandate. For the purposes of this book, these categories are described hereafter as *proximal principals* and *distal principals*. As these titles imply, they suggest that the IO perceives its relationship with various principals differently. While all the WHO's member states form one collective body, proximal principals are those member states that the WHO has *collectively* determined are critical to its overall mission, due to either the normative or material support of its mandate. Particular care is usually taken not to offend or unduly antagonize proximal principals due to their perceived strategic importance and/or influence.[2] Distal principals, by way of contrast, are those member states that the WHO collectively fails to hold in high esteem, or holds fragmented views about (see ibid., pp. 370–2), either because they do not appear to take an active interest in or oversight of the IO's activities, or because their influence and/or material support of the organization is minimal.

In the context of the WHO, PA theory thus offers a valuable framework for analysing the IO secretariat's adoption of security-related terminology and concepts given the objections that a number of countries have raised. Is this an instance of agency slack? To what extent is the secretariat's adoption of this agenda consistent with the IO's mandate, purpose, and function? Given that only a few member states have apparently voiced objections to the WHO's health security agenda, does this constitute a breach of the secretariat's powers and authority?

The following work will engage with these questions and seek to provide some definitive answers.

The second analytical framework that has been used to evaluate the WHO's actions draws on the Copenhagen School's securitization theory (Buzan et al. 1998). In their work, Buzan and his colleagues set out to 'explore the logic of security itself to find out what differentiates security . . . from that which is merely political' (ibid., p. 5). This is because the successful invocation of 'security' in relation to a particular issue or subject changes the nature of political discourse, moving the issue outside of the realm of normal political debate. Security 'takes politics beyond the established rules of the game and frames the issue either as a special kind of politics or as above politics' (ibid., p. 23). This elevated political state in turn permits – and at times even necessitates – that exceptional measures be taken because security 'means survival in the face of existential threats' (ibid., p. 27). Said another way, '[an] issue becomes a security issue . . . not necessarily because a real existential threat exists but because the issue is presented as a threat' (ibid., p. 24). Buzan and his colleagues describe the process by which this occurs as securitization – the intentional utilization of speech acts by securitizing actors to evoke and convey to a target audience a sense of grave vulnerability, thereby provoking an endorsement of exceptional measures from that audience to address the issue (McDonald 2008, p. 567, Balzacq 2011, p. 3). Accordingly, there are three critical components to successful securitization: (i) a securitizing move (i.e. speech act), (ii) securitizing actors, and (iii) an audience that has the ability to authorize exceptional measures.

Three further points are important at this juncture. While much has been made of the Copenhagen School's securitization treatise within security studies literature, it is equally important to remember that securitization is ultimately a framing exercise (Watson 2012). The use of frames (framing) as tools whereby particular actors (agents) apply pressure on decision-makers to affect public policy has been analysed extensively throughout a variety of fields, including psychology, media studies, linguistics, sociology, and political studies (Benford and Snow 2000). Frames can take a variety of forms (i.e. linguistic, cognitive, cultural, symbolic), but are deployed in order to provide 'conceptual coherence, a direction for action, a basis for persuasion, and a framework for the collection and analysis of data' (Rein and Schön 1993, p. 153). Framing exercises can thereby be distinguished from simple persuasion, which, as Nelson and Oxley (1999, p. 1041) have suggested, occurs when someone 'effectively revises the content of one's beliefs about the attitude object, replacing or supplementing favourable thoughts with unfavourable ones, or vice versa'. By way of contrast, while frames 'may affect the content of one's beliefs, they also affect the *importance* individuals attach to particular beliefs' (ibid., p. 1041, italics original). In so doing, agents use frames to highlight and confer legitimacy upon particular facets of reality while side-lining other elements (Lawrence 2000). Moreover, a 'successful framing exercise will both cause an issue to be seen by those that matter, and ensure that they see it in a particular way' (Bøås and McNeill 2004, p. 1).

In many regards, the relationship between frames and public policy is best viewed as mutually constitutive. That is to say, as much as frames may be used (intentionally or otherwise) to affect public policy, such policies equally 'rest on frames that supply them with underlying structures of beliefs, perception, and appreciation' (Fischer 2003, p. 144). Seen in this light, public policy changes occur when one set of frames is replaced by another set of more convincing metaphors, axioms, allegories, symbols, and images. Critical to any framing activity, however, is the role of agency – in both developing and deploying the frame(s) as well as the audience to whom the frame(s) are directed (namely decision-makers, general public, etc). For not only do policy entrepreneurs engage in re-framing exercises to advance new policy outcomes or to overcome situations whereby conflicting frames have paralysed decision-making processes (ibid.), but as Nelson (2004, p. 584) has gone on to observe, 'Successful frames must consider the target audience's existing values and emphasize the special importance of a particular value for a given issue, rather than infuse the audience with an entirely new value structure'.

An additional caveat to note is that whereas Buzan and colleagues argue that there are three critical components to successful securitization (a securitizing move, securitizing actors, and an audience), this work insists that a fourth factor – context – is also essential. In this, the following investigation aligns more closely with the sociological view of securitization theory advanced by Balzacq (2011) and others. Said another way, securitization has often been portrayed as a relatively straight-forward process in which securitizing actor(s) engage in securitizing move(s) that then convince target audience(s) of peril to endorse exceptional measures. What is often neglected within this narrative, however, is an analysis of the context in which such a process occurs. This is an important factor as the socio-economic, political, and cultural context will affect not only how the message is structured and communicated, but also how it is received, ultimately determining whether securitization is successful (Salter 2008). While some post-structuralist scholars maintain that Balzacq's (2011) work is flawed, as context is always embedded within securitizing moves (i.e. discourse) (Hansen 2011), highlighting context as a distinct factor is nevertheless useful as an analytical tool for unpacking power imbalances and subtleties – and indeed this is perhaps even more critical in the complex relationship environment that exists between principals and their agents.

For many IR theorists, the attempt to integrate PA theory and the Copenhagen School's securitization theory will be controversial. This is principally because it is often held that rationalist and constructivist approaches are diametrically opposed. This book rejects such arguments though, and in this regard aligns more closely with the work of Oestreich (2012) and Graham (2014) who have similarly sought to integrate rationalist and constructivist accounts when interpreting the behaviour of IOs. Oestreich and colleagues quite convincingly argue that constructivist and rationalist theories can actually complement each other by providing a framework whereby PA theory facilitates testable hypotheses regarding preference homo- and heterogeneity and the ability to interrogate how agents attempt to slip or shirk their obligations, while constructivist approaches allow for the possibility that interests may change, thereby allowing greater opportunity to examine the internal processes within organizations. Oestreich (2012, p.11) argues that the combination of these two approaches 'tells us something about what IOs actually do with their independence, not just from where that independence comes'. Drawing on the earlier work of Cox and Jacobsen (1973), Oestreich (2012, p. 15) goes on to argue that IOs may be assessed as 'acting' when they both exhibit independence in addition to having a discernible impact on outcomes. As the remainder of this book seeks to outline in some depth, the WHO has displayed considerable independence in advancing the global health security narrative, which in turn has had an evident impact on how governments and even other IOs have approached hazards to human health.

It would also be prudent at this stage to say a few words about what is meant by *managing* global health security. As noted above, how global health security is conceptualized and viewed has changed and expanded in recent years. Although there still remains some conjecture over how to define the term (see Aldis 2008, McInnes 2015), as Rushton (2012, p. 782) has noted there nevertheless appears to be general consensus over the 'core features' of health security, particularly in terms of the types of health issues that constitute a threat (i.e. infectious diseases and weaponized pathogens), what comprises legitimate and appropriate responses (i.e. government-led), and the referent object (i.e. the state). The WHO has a critical administrative role to play within each of these three areas, but the nature of that role, and the authority that the organization is ostensibly permitted to exercise, is also slightly different in each context. In terms of the threat, for instance, as will be explored in greater detail in Chapter One, the WHO's primary mission is to prevent, wherever possible, the emergence of epidemics and pandemics, and when they do occur, to play *the* lead role in overseeing and directing international efforts to safeguard human health. At the same time, that authority is not unbridled, but is in fact subject to a raft of checks and balances. In responding to disease outbreaks, epidemics, and pandemics the WHO does not, for example, possess the authority to intervene in the domestic affairs of individual member states, except by invitation. The organization's role is instead relegated to more of an advisory function, issuing recommendations on what governments can (and should) do to mitigate the event but possessing no powers or authority to compel. It is in this context that the WHO's constituents are, first and foremost, its member states (i.e. governments) as opposed to the peoples of the world, and it is answerable to those governments for the actions it does, or does not, take. The term 'manage' has thereby been used purposefully to describe the distinct types of authority that the WHO utilizes in different circumstances and environments, ranging from oversight and coordination to physical/practical interventions wherever need exists and is permitted.

What, however, is the WHO managing? As will become evident in the following pages, the definition of global health security applied throughout this book pertains to the mitigation of fast moving, acute hazards to human health arising from infectious diseases. While some may view this as an unduly narrow interpretation that is no longer reflective of the wider emergent field of inquiry, as this book explicitly argues, the control and eradication of infectious diseases has been the central feature of the WHO's existence since its founding. While the motivations for why the IO pursued the elimination of infectious diseases may have been amended slightly over time, like Rushton (2012) this book maintains that there is in fact considerable consensus about the phrase and its associated concept.

In light of this, it is also worthwhile to spend a few moments delineating what is meant when referring to 'the World Health Organization'. The WHO was created in 1948 as the first specialized agency of the UN, and as such, its structure and organizational design broadly reflects that of its parent institution. Indeed, like the UN, the WHO is comprised of three organs: the World Health Assembly (WHA), an Executive Board (EB), and a secretariat, which includes the director-general. The WHA, which is equivalent to the UN General Assembly and comprised solely of member states, serves as the ultimate decision-making body determining the organization's policies, programmes, and budget. The EB is similar in some respects to the Security Council of the UN in that it is comprised of a smaller sub-set of representatives (currently 34 technically qualified individuals) who, although appointed by governments, were originally intended to serve in their capacity as independent experts overseeing the work of the organization and ensuring that the bureaucratic arm of the institution is performing as directed. The WHO's third organ – the secretariat – consists of the director-general, who serves as the organization's chief technical officer, and a staff of professionally qualified personnel to execute the directives of the WHA. At the time of writing, the secretariat comprises approximately 8,000 employees divided between the organization's central headquarters in Geneva, Switzerland, six regional offices, and 142 country offices. For the purposes of this book, therefore, whenever 'the WHO' or 'the organization' is used it is intended to refer explicitly to the administrative element, or bureaucracy, of the intergovernmental organization. This specifically comprises the Office of the Director-General (including the director-general herself), the secretariat, and the Executive Board, which maintains oversight of the secretariat and is predominantly comprised of technical experts. Unless otherwise expressly indicated, the WHA is excluded from the definition of the WHO used throughout this book and will be treated as a distinct entity. This is principally because the WHA consists of the appointed representatives of 194 member states, and as such very little distinction can be drawn between the WHA and the governments of the world.

Indeed, it is important to recall that when discussing IOs and evaluating their work, it is actually the actions of people that are being assessed. As Oestreich (2012, p. 13) has noted, 'IOs are comprised of people' and 'to understand the activities of IOs we must know something of the people within them'. The ideas and beliefs that people hold influence their actions, and particularly where there is a preponderance of like-minded individuals (i.e. professionals such as medical doctors), those ideas can have a significant impact upon the direction of an organization. It is in this regard that in analysing the evolution of the WHO's policies and practices towards preventing, controlling, and eliminating diseases that considerable attention is also given to the role of certain individuals within the WHO at particular points in time, especially if they held (or still hold) senior positions of authority. By taking this dual approach of examining the context in which decisions are made and the role that specific individuals played within that environment, the book hopes to avoid the well-trodden debate within IR about agency versus structure. Both are important for the simple fact that when artificially separated and examined independently, neither can fully explain the complex, multifaceted world in which we live.

Further, it is important to note that less attention has been afforded to the role of the WHO's member states in the following analysis than perhaps what some might expect or wish to see. This is for two primary reasons. First, as noted earlier, this book has as its focus a series of inter-related objectives that includes highlighting the significance of the WHO, the evolution of the organization's approach to managing global health security, and the influence of certain ideas, values, and beliefs in shaping communicable disease-related global health policy. As such, attention is only given to the role of member states where there is evidence of a clear and discernible impact on the WHO's health security mission, as otherwise it will serve to distract from these objectives.

The second justification for why so little attention has been given to the impact of particular governments is that, as noted above, the WHA currently consists of 194 countries. Conducting a survey of 194 governments in relation to each shift or turn in the WHO's policies would be impracticable for one relatively modest-sized monograph; moreover, like IOs, even individual countries exist as *societies of societies* – a conglomeration of self-constituting collectives of human beings (Barberis 2003). Gauging the views of any one country at a particular point in time thereby becomes particularly problematic, let alone the collective position of 194 countries, as people's views and beliefs can change from moment to moment. Where the official positions of governments can be seen to have had a direct bearing on the WHO's approach to global health security, they are appropriately noted, but equally it must be recalled that the WHA operates on a 'one country, one vote' system, which means that – at least officially – no one individual country has greater sway than another. For these reasons, less attention has been given to identifying the role and impact of individual countries and how they may, or may not, have influenced events.

Before going on to examine the origins of the WHO (Chapter One), it is also necessary to say a few words about the case studies used in this book, and specifically the absence of any analysis surrounding the governance of HIV/AIDS. The emergence of HIV/AIDS in the 1980s and its progressive spread around the world arguably exists as one of the most devastating events in the history of global public health (Piot 2006). The disease has killed millions of people, and despite billions of dollars being spent in establishing prevention and treatment programmes, every year millions more are infected. Given this reality, and the fact that a core focus of this book is examining global communicable disease health policy, it would be reasonable to expect some discussion and engagement with the global governance of HIV/AIDS. Importantly, however, very little discussion or analysis of this specific disease has been included in this volume for two chief reasons.

The first is that responsibility for responding to the HIV/AIDS crisis has been devolved to multiple global governance institutions and is no longer the exclusive domain of the WHO. In fact, the WHO is only one of several key institutions that contribute to global HIV/AIDS policy. In large part, this outcome is a direct consequence of the WHO's gross mishandling of the HIV/AIDS crisis in the 1990s that resulted, amongst other things, in the creation of an entirely new, purpose-built IO – the Joint United Nations Programme on HIV/AIDS (UNAIDS) (Fee and Parry 2008). In addition, as the pandemic has continued to grow, so too has recognition of the multi-dimensional nature of the disease and its impact on various sectors of society. This in turn has prompted the involvement of other non-health global governance institutions such as the World Bank, the International Monetary Fund (IMF), the G8, and the G20, as well as the creation of multiple global health partnerships such as the Global Fund for HIV/AIDS, Tuberculosis, and Malaria ('the Global Fund'), UNITAID, and the H8 ('Health 8', an informal group of eight *health*-related organizations), to name just a few. As noted earlier, however, the focus of this book is on the WHO's health security policies and procedures, noting how they have changed and adapted over time. Although the WHO continues to remain actively engaged in the governance of HIV/AIDS, the organization's earlier mismanagement and the extrication of this specific disease to another purpose-built IO disqualify its evaluation and assessment here.

The second, related reason for why so little attention is accorded to HIV/AIDS in this book is that the vast majority of existing GHG literature already tends to focus overwhelmingly on HIV/AIDS. Accordingly, there are several works already in existence that more adequately and comprehensively engage not only with the global governance of HIV/AIDS (see, for example, Hein et al. 2007, Poku et al. 2007, Harman and Lisk 2009), but also with the security implications and/or securitization of the disease (Elbe 2003, 2006, 2009, Aginam and Rupiya 2012, Rushton 2012, Seckinelgin 2012). For these reasons, there is clearly less need to devote much time or attention to discussing the WHO's involvement in the global governance of HIV/AIDS in any great depth, as the topic has been sufficiently covered elsewhere.

Structure of the book

The book has been structured into three parts, with two chapters forming each part. Part I is concerned with establishing the WHO's delegated authority for managing global health security and how that authority had traditionally been exercised. Accordingly, Chapter One examines the constitutional powers of the WHO for controlling and eradicating infectious diseases, and the limitations that member states have imposed on that authority through various legal, financial, and technical means. Chapter Two then examines how the IO sought to demonstrate its authority through various disease eradication initiatives. Accordingly, the chapter surveys three case studies – the Malaria Eradication Programme (MEP), the Smallpox Eradication Programme (SEP), and the WHO's efforts to eliminate tuberculosis (TB). These three case studies have been chosen principally to highlight how the WHO progressively developed a conventional approach to disease control and eradication. The MEP has been selected, for example, as it served as the WHO's first-ever attempt at completely eradicating an infectious disease, but for various reasons explored in the chapter the programme proved unsuccessful. By way of contrast, the WHO's success in eradicating smallpox is frequently hailed as the IO's greatest public health achievement. Importantly, however, both these programmes were massive global eradication campaigns that attracted significant resources and support. As such, the WHO's programme to eliminate TB as a public health menace has also been selected to juxtapose the MEP and SEP. The WHO's efforts to control TB also serves as a helpful case study as it is the only instance prior to the 2003 SARS outbreak where the IO declared the spread of one specific disease a global public health emergency. When collectively viewed, these case studies reveal that the WHO had developed a standard or classical approach to controlling and eliminating infectious diseases in which the IO functioned largely as a coordinating authority, eschewing its ability to direct the international community's responses due to past failures and concerns that it would result in further constraints being imposed on the IO.

In Part II, the book explores the period that led to the WHO's adoption of security-related concepts and language to fulfil its duty of eradicating infectious diseases. Chapter Three therefore examines the IO's securitization of infectious diseases and its management of the 2003 SARS outbreak. Indeed, the WHO's management of SARS marked a distinct turning point in the organization's approach to global health security, allowing the IO to test a variety of new techniques and methods that ultimately proved so successful that they served to reinvigorate the IO's reputation and international standing. The WHO's management of SARS subsequently informed the final stages of the International Health Regulations (IHR) revision process – the focus of Chapter Four – that had originally begun in 1995 following a series of events that highlighted the WHO's traditional approach to controlling and eliminating infectious diseases was insufficient. Importantly, however, as this chapter goes on to explore, some of the exceptional measures taken by the secretariat, and the ease with which it did so, concerned the IO's principals to the extent that, in the final stages of the IHR revision process, they sought to reign in the organization's powers by inserting new legal constraints and technical requirements on the IO's delegation contract.

Part III of the book then examines the WHO's management of global health security post-SARS. Specifically, Chapter Five investigates the WHO's response to the emergence and progressive spread of the H5N1 avian influenza 'bird flu' virus, the organization's response to the 2009 H1N1 influenza 'swine flu' pandemic, and the controversies that arose surrounding its management of this event. Chapter Six then explores the criticisms that have emerged of the WHO's securitization of certain select health issues, and how the IO has reacted to these events and the much closer scrutiny of member states by now downplaying the health-as-security discourse. Using the WHO's management of recent public health crises, the chapter also discusses what the future of the IO's approach to managing global health security may look like. The book then concludes by returning to the theoretical considerations with a short discussion and evaluation of what these current trends suggest about IO pathology, desecuritization, and the future of the WHO as it seeks to fulfil its disease eradication mandate.

1
The Legal Basis for the WHO's Global Health Security Mandate and Authority

In 1946 when the WHO's constitution was written, some 22 functions and duties were ascribed to the organization. Of these, the WHO's chief function is the control and eradication of infectious diseases. Although often unspoken, the priority attached to this particular task is understandable when reviewing the historical origins of the WHO and the events of the immediate post-war period. The focus of this chapter is to outline the WHO's delegated authority for eradicating infectious diseases, noting the terms and limitations of that authority, and the mechanisms by which member states have sought to exercise control over the IO to prevent agency slack. The chapter will also survey the historical origins of the WHO, with a particular focus on identifying the key ideas that both informed and shaped its creation and overall mandate. This chapter thereby establishes the foundation upon which the rest of the book is based, as it is only from an understanding of this delegated authority that we can, firstly, appreciate why so much importance has been assigned to this one central task, and secondly, understand why the organization's approach to managing global health security has changed and adapted over time.

Said another way, the WHO has a legal obligation to its member states to assist them in responding to, controlling, and ideally eliminating infectious diseases. This obligation was established by what international law describes as a 'delegation of powers' from member states to an IO (Sarooshi 2005), and results in what PA theorists describe as a 'delegation contract' (Hawkins et al. 2006). As discussed in the Introduction, it was originally intended that the WHO would act as the directing and coordinating authority in all international health matters (and particularly in eradicating infectious diseases), actively guiding the international community's efforts (Mackenzie 1950). Even so, the methods that the organization's secretariat has used at times to pursue this mandate have attracted some controversy. For example, in the midst of the SARS-inspired global emergency in 2003, questions were raised over the extent of the IO's role and authority (Rodier 2003). Some even suggested that the organization's director-general and secretariat exceeded their authority, that they exercised 'independent power' (agency slack), and that in doing so the WHO's bureaucracy had brought about a new era of 'post-Westphalian' health governance (Fidler 2004, Cortell and Peterson 2006). Questions were also raised in the aftermath of the 2009 H1N1 influenza pandemic, although attention then focused on the role that pharmaceutical companies had played in the director-general's decision to declare a pandemic (Godlee 2010). While a number of internal and external investigations were launched to evaluate the WHO's actions – with every investigation subsequently absolving the secretariat of any wrongdoing – it is evident that many of the policies and procedures the IO uses to pursue its health security mandate are not clearly understood. Where does the organization derive its authority? What is the extent of these powers? To fully appreciate this, we need first to examine the historical origins of the WHO.

The WHO's historical origins and ethos

The creation of the WHO as a new intergovernmental organization dedicated to improving the world's health reflected a particular world-view of the post-war period. This worldview held that IOs were an important mechanism for arranging international society to prevent further conflict. In this, the work of David Mitrany proved particularly influential in the closing months of the second, most destructive war humanity had ever known (Ashworth 2005, Fidler and Gostin 2008). Mitrany postulated that one of the principal causes of conflict was 'the baffling division between the peoples of the world' into nation-states, as they encouraged the emergence of nationalism, which served to divide rather than unite populations (Mitrany 1946, p. 5). To overcome this problem and thereby prevent further war, Mitrany advocated that inter-national society needed to be re-arranged along functional lines and serviced by independent, apolitical, technical organizations. The central premise of his treatise was that the nation-state was redundant, as it was incapable of providing the requisite physical, social, and economic security to its citizens due to transnational forces beyond the control of any one government. Arguing that peoples' loyalty to the state was integrally linked with the provision of services, Mitrany suggested that if IOs assumed these functions, then the citizens' loyalty to the state would correspondingly shift. As the needs of populations were being met by IOs, people would increasingly see themselves less as citizens of individual countries and more as 'citizens of the world'. Circumventing any concerns that he was advocating some form of Communist revolution, Mitrany also argued that this transition could be accomplished peacefully and incrementally: governments did not have to surrender their sovereignty, but rather progressively delegate responsibility for the provision of services to purpose-built IOs designed to meet specific social and economic needs. This functional approach to world order, the theory held, thus avoided the divisive competition for resources and the negative influence of politics, as peoples' needs were met by functional, technical organizations.

Given the political climate of the post-World War II (WWII) period and his intimate involvement in post-war reconstruction efforts (Ashworth 1999), Mitrany's functional approach to world politics garnered widespread support. The philosophical basis of Mitrany's argument – that further conflict could be avoided through independent, apolitical IOs meeting peoples' needs – appealed to many wearied by war. Functionalism, as Mitrany's theory subsequently became known, came to be viewed as a legitimate political theory of International Organization and was heavily influential in the development of the UN and its specialized agencies such as the United Nations Educational, Scientific and Cultural Organization (UNESCO) and the WHO (Haas 1956, Siddiqi 1995). Moreover, although criticisms of this approach continue to emerge (Davis 2012), the philosophical underpinnings of functionalism – that the provision of certain services can be extricated from compromising political interference, thereby averting conflict – remains a guiding force in contemporary IO practice (Hale and Held 2012).

In the specific context of health, Mitrany's proposal for technocratic, apolitical IOs to deliver specific services corresponded with two other developments that had been growing in popularity: the concept of health as a civil right and the rise of social medicine. The idea that health was every citizen's entitlement and an obligation of the state had been gaining strength throughout the 19th century. Importantly, however, the primary focus of government-led initiatives during this period had been on preventing epidemics, and very few countries had instituted any widespread, state-sponsored programmes designed to improve overall population health. At the end of World War I (WWI) though, this situation changed dramatically as countries throughout Europe and the Americas instigated various initiatives to redress the massive loss of human life brought about by The Great War. Programmes focusing on eugenics as well as maternal and child health became standard, but expectations surrounding the role of the state in the provision of health and medical services did not ultimately come to the fore until towards the end of WWII (Porter 1999).

Likewise, although social medicine had its origins in the late 19th century, throughout the interwar years it had come to be increasingly recognized that factors such as housing, income, food quality, and the like had a discernible impact on population health and well-being. In contrast to clinical medicine – which focused on rectifying faults in the human body via surgical intervention or the burgeoning field of pharmacology – social medicine promoted the idea that achieving good health could only be realized by addressing the social and economic inequalities that contributed to ill health. The social medicine movement thereby adopted an explicit political agenda that both coincided with and argued in support of welfare provision and social security – themes that received considerable support in a post-war environment. As a concept and practice, social medicine then gained yet further support throughout the interwar years due to the fact that several of the world's then-leading health experts – many of whom held prominent positions within governments and international institutions – actively endorsed its implementation (Porter 2006). Thus, despite the fact that the return of hostilities in 1939 impeded progress in advancing the social medicine agenda for a time, the foundations for the movement's influence in future international health cooperation had nevertheless been laid.

Indeed, in the closing months of WWII addressing social and economic disparities and ensuring sufficient levels of social security were viewed with an additional level of significance. By 1945 it had come to be widely accepted that the reparations imposed on Germany by the Treaty of Versailles in 1919 had caused massive social and economic disruption, which in turn had generated significant discontent amongst the segment of Germany's population that aided the rise of the Nazi regime to power (Lauterbach 1944, Klein 1948). For many involved in post-war reconstruction efforts, a clear link therefore existed between social welfare provision and international security. Health and access to healthcare services subsequently came to be viewed as integral to not only ensuring domestic stability but also to enabling international peace and security. Health was viewed as a means to peace and was seen as just one area in which technical cooperation (such as that championed by Mitrany's functional approach) could flourish.

It is in this regard that the connections between health, international security, and the WHO can be traced back to the origins of the organization. From its very founding, a strong correlation existed between the idea that international security was attained and maintained by ensuring good health, and it was expected that governments would cooperate to protect the peace that had been so hard won. Having said this, the correlations between health and security as conceived in the immediate post-war period contrasts significantly with the health-security nexus of the 21st century. Whereas post-WWII good health was deemed essential to maintaining peace and security – resulting in the outlook of health-for-security – by the turn of the new millennium (and as subsequent chapters go on to explore), the focus had inverted, so that health had become synonymous with security – or health-as-security.

The decision taken in 1946 to create a new, universal health agency epitomized the functional approach to world politics, but also reflected dissatisfaction with the existing intergovernmental institutions responsible for the control of infectious disease.[1] The adverse effect that disease outbreaks could have on international trade (and thereby on national economic interests) had long been recognized by governments. In the 14th century the city-state of Venice was the first to institute a system of quarantine designed to protect its inhabitants from diseases aboard ships travelling along international trade routes. Within a matter of years, other European authorities instituted their own versions of quarantine, but significant inconsistencies existed between them, due in large part to differing beliefs about how diseases spread (Porter 1999). In an attempt to limit the negative impact that varying quarantine practices were having on international trade, the first International Sanitary Conference was convened in Paris in 1851. The conference lasted a full six months, and although the delegates of the 12 countries in attendance agreed to a set of regulations comprising 137 articles, all except two governments failed to ratify the agreement (WHO 1958).[2] Between 1851 and 1938, a further 15 conferences and meetings were convened (often in direct response to an epidemic that was then sweeping throughout Europe) in an attempt to overcome the differences between countries. Yet while authorities failed in their objective of developing a consistent system of measures, the repeated epidemics of cholera, plague, typhoid, and yellow fever, amongst other diseases, emphasized the need for greater international coordination and cooperation (Goodman 1952).

Accordingly, in 1907 the Office Internationale d'Hygiene Publique (OIHP) was founded in Paris, France, by the League of Red Cross Societies to monitor the emergence and spread of disease outbreaks. One of the key tasks assigned to the OIHP was to gather and interpret epidemiological data, which it would then publish in a weekly journal. Yet while the OIHP performed its duties perfunctorily, the organization was widely perceived as being concerned exclusively with affairs that affected Europe – a perception aided by the fact the IO only ever published its findings in the French language. It thus emerged that following the creation of the League of Nations at the end of WWI, in 1922 a decision was taken to establish a health division of the League that would adopt a wider focus in addressing the widespread famine and disease that had emerged in the aftermath of the war. The League of Nations Health Organization (LNHO) was created the following year (LNHO 1931). Yet while the LNHO engendered greater support than its parent organization, like the League it failed to secure North American participation and was thereby unable to claim universal membership. Rather than stimulate cooperation, however, the relationship between the OIHP and LNHO became marred by controversy and competition (Howard-Jones 1978). Added to this, various regional organizations such as the Pan American Sanitary Organization (PASO) (which later was renamed the Pan American Health Organization [PAHO] in 1958) and the Pan Arab Regional Health Bureau further complicated the jurisdictional boundaries. In 1943, fearing a repeat of the various epidemics that arose at the end of WWI, the international health sphere became even further complicated by the creation of the United Nations Relief and Rehabilitation Administration (UNRRA), which was built specifically to help liberated populations recover and rebuild as soon as possible. Addressing health needs, including preventing disease outbreaks, epidemics, and pandemics, was a core focus of the UNRRA's work (Goodman 1952). As a result of this complex environment, by the end of WWII there was broad agreement that the existing institutions should be subsumed within a new universal agency – a new world health organization – to ensure more effective international cooperation (Sharp 1947).

Given this history, it is understandable that several of these prevailing ideas and beliefs would inform the development of the WHO. Reflecting the contemporary view that health was a civil right, for example, the preamble of the new IO's constitution explicitly declared that 'enjoyment of the highest attainable standard of health is one of the fundamental rights of every human being' (Preamble, WHO Constitution – WHO 2005a, p. 1). Evidencing the conviction that the provision of social welfare was integral to ensuring a conflict-free world, the constitution was drafted to note that the health 'of all peoples is fundamental to the attainment of peace and security' (ibid.). Finally, exemplifying the broader principles of social medicine, the Constitution specified that health was defined as 'a state of complete physical, mental and social well-being and not merely the absence of disease or infirmity' and that 'Governments have a responsibility for the health of their peoples which can be fulfilled only by the provision of adequate health and social measures' (ibid.).

To facilitate the merger of multiple organizations into a single entity, the Interim Commission of the World Health Organization was formed in 1946 to oversee the transition. It took almost a full two years before the requisite 26th member state ratified the WHO Constitution on 7 April 1948, officially establishing the new IO. As one commentator later recorded though, 'For all practical purposes, and despite this dilatoriness of governments . . . WHO had existed since 1946' (Calder 1958, p. 5). Indeed, the Commission immediately set about adopting the work of the OIHP, the UNRRA, and the now largely defunct LNHO in gathering epidemiological intelligence and responding to disease-related emergencies while also initiating negotiations with the PASO to integrate the regional organization within the WHO. These discussions took the better part of three years to conclude before the PASO became the WHO's regional office for the Americas on 1 July 1949 (WHO 1958).

Importantly, however, the negotiations surrounding the integration of the PASO also had a wider effect in determining the overall structure and operation of the new WHO. The International Sanitary Bureau had been originally established in 1902 by the US government to help overcome 'the complicated mosaic of differing quarantine, inspection, and exclusion regulations that impeded the movement of goods' throughout the Americas (Fee and Brown 2002, p. 1888). The Bureau, which was renamed the Pan American Sanitary Bureau (PASB) in 1923, then joined with the Pan American Sanitary Conferences in 1947 to become the PASO. Critically, throughout its existence the organization had retained an explicit regional focus on the Americas – a focus that the leaders of the PASB/PASO were reluctant to surrender. Accordingly, when the proposal to create a single new universal health agency was made in 1946, the PASB campaigned fiercely to retain its independence from the WHO (Lee 2009). Eventually, a compromise deal was struck in 1949 that permitted the now PASO to become the WHO's regional office for the Americas, with autonomy over its own budget and programme of work (Sharp 1947, Fee and Brown 2002, Burci and Vignes 2004). The precedent established by the PASO, however, permitted other regions to argue for equivalent arrangements, with the result that by 1951 some six regional offices had been created – the Americas, the Western Pacific,

South-East Asia, the Middle East, Europe, and Africa – overseen by a central headquarters based in Geneva, Switzerland. This arrangement has subsequently led some to argue that there is not one WHO but rather seven organizations (six regional offices and a central headquarters), which contributes to a raft of inefficiencies, duplication of services, and poor health outcomes (Godlee 1994, WHO 1999a, Burci and Vignes 2004, p. 121). Equally though, on the converse side, the autonomy granted to the regional offices has also ensured that they are more readily able to target the diverse health needs of member states' populations. This arrangement thereby facilitates a closer relationship between the WHO and its member states, with the latter dictating how and where the organization is authorized to assist.

Disease eradication and the envisaged authority of the WHO

For the WHO secretariat, pursuing the prevention, control, and eradication of infectious diseases is a fundamental obligation. This is perhaps no more clearly articulated than in Article 2 of the WHO Constitution, which states that the organization is required 'to stimulate and advance work to eradicate epidemic, endemic and other diseases' (WHO 2005a, p. 2). However, the organization's duty to pursue the goal of disease eradication has also been repeatedly stressed by member states through a series of WHA resolutions, through several other references and provisions throughout the WHO Constitution, and through dedicated international framework agreements such as the IHR and the 2011 PIP Framework. When collectively viewed, these documents (and the stipulations they contain therein) form the basis of an embedded *disease eradication delegation contract* between the IO and its member states.

The contract as it currently exists, however, is a very fluid, and in some ways intangible pact. It is not possible, for instance, to point to one specific document that comprehensively delineates the parameters of the organization's disease eradication responsibilities, obligations, or powers. Rather, as indicated above, the contract comprises a series of provisions and stipulations that are contained within three distinct sets of documents. Each collection of these documents serves to establish, expand, and/or reduce the WHO's delegated contractual obligations in responding to and managing infectious disease outbreaks. It also is in this regard that the 'contract' has continued to evolve, expand, and adapt over time as WHA resolutions, revisions to existing and/or the creation of new treaties and regulations, and new operational practices have altered the nature and terms of the original contract.

One of the key milestones in the development of the WHO's disease eradication mandate was the passage of the International Sanitary Regulations (ISR) in 1951. Following the inability of the International Sanitary Conferences to arrive at a uniform set of measures to prevent disease outbreaks and epidemics severely disrupting international trade, the Interim Commission of the WHO was charged with this task when it was created in 1946. Work to develop a universal agreement began in earnest in 1948, and on 25 May 1951 the Fourth WHA passed the *WHA4.75 WHO Regulations No.2, the International Sanitary Regulations* resolution (Burci and Vignes 2004, p. 135). The passage of this resolution marked an important landmark in the history of infectious disease control, finally achieving an objective that had begun a full century earlier. Equally though, the adoption of this one resolution signalled an important development in expanding and clarifying the WHO's disease eradication responsibilities.

The ISR, which were later renamed the IHR in 1969, established a framework for cooperation that the WHO's member states and the IO's bureaucracy could follow in the event of an international disease outbreak. Drafted specifically to address the menace presented by six 'notifiable' diseases – cholera, plague, typhus, smallpox, yellow fever, and relapsing fever – the Regulations required member states to abide by a set of prescriptions and recommendations designed to prevent the importation of these diseases (WHO 1951). Yet despite their relatively limited scope – which by 1981 had been progressively reduced even further to cover only three diseases (cholera, plague, and yellow fever) – since their inception the ISR/IHR were beset with problems associated with member states' non-compliance and under-reporting (Delon 1975). The challenges associated with IHR non-compliance and evasion eventually prompted the WHA, in 1995, to order that they be updated and revised (see Chapter Four). Even so, the passage of a purpose-built framework just three years after the WHO had been created established the broad parameters for how member states were expected to behave when confronted with the international spread of disease, while also serving to reinforce the WHO's disease control and eradication credentials in ensuring health-for-security.

At this juncture, however, it is important to pause for a moment to stress that the WHO's disease eradication duties have always extended beyond the notifiable diseases. For example, as will become apparent in the next chapter, the WHO has been involved in the control and elimination of TB since its inception, yet TB has never been listed amongst those diseases requiring notification. Similarly, the emergence of HIV/AIDS in the early 1980s technically existed beyond the scope of the ISR/IHR, yet member states have readily accepted that the organization has a key role to play in working towards the eradication of that disease. By and large, governments the world over have correspondingly reported their respective national prevalence rates to the IO and accepted its technical guidance on the matter (WHO 2014a). It is in this regard that the contract is perhaps best viewed as dynamic and fluid, as two additional factors – WHA resolutions and new practices – have also had a significant influence on the scope and extent of the overall agreement that grants the WHO its powers.

WHA resolutions form an integral component of the WHO's disease eradication delegation contract. By their very nature, resolutions passed by a simple majority of member states are legally binding on the organization's bureaucracy. They may therefore serve to augment or narrow the IO's contract, placing new restrictions on the WHO's autonomy, authority, and competence, or conversely, by expanding the capacity of the organization's operational activities respectively. Accordingly, the WHO's ability to execute its disease eradication function has changed over time as member states have attached greater significance to the control and/ or eradication of some communicable disease threats over others.

Likewise, the practices of the WHO have also had a notable effect on the IO's disease eradication delegation contract. Within the legal sphere, this is what is known as customary international law (Cassese 2005), and IOs, like states, are deemed competent to provide new interpretations of international law through their actions (Alvarez 2005). In the context of the WHO, as the organization has pursued its duty to eradicate diseases, the outworking or manifestation of that authority has served to shape and manipulate the nature, essence, and extent of its delegated responsibilities. Through interaction with member states and by determining what methods/actions are acceptable and permissible, new interpretations have arisen regarding the WHO's role, authority, and autonomy within the contract. It is in this regard that the contract has been influenced by the IO's praxis or customs.

It has occasionally been suggested, however, that the WHO accords far too much attention to infectious diseases, paying insufficient consideration to other health issues such as non-communicable disease (Bale 2002, Banerjee 2010). On the surface this conclusion may initially appear sound, given that the WHO Constitution lists the WHO's disease eradication function as only one obligation amongst some 21 further assigned functions. In addition, various commentators have also suggested that the functions cited in Article 2 of the Constitution appear randomly, in no order of importance or priority (Burci and Vignes 2004,

p. 119). Given these observations, it would be reasonable to surmise that the WHO is expected to grant equal attention to all 22 functions, fulfilling them all without prejudice (WHO 1948a). Yet as any review of the WHO's programmes and activities will reveal, the organization's bureaucracy has failed to do so. Is this therefore a case of IO agency slippage? Or is it possible that another explanation may account for this apparent discrepancy? Three further points are warranted here.

As noted above, health was defined by the founders of the WHO to be a state of complete physical, mental, and social well-being and not merely the absence of disease or infirmity. This definition has attracted considerable controversy over the years, primarily because it advocates a wider, holistic view than most biomedical or clinical medicine conceptualizations of health. Those who decry the WHO's definition often point to the elusive or ethereal nature of mental and social well-being and the corresponding inability to measure or quantify what 'good' health would look like, while those who champion the IO's broader view of health argue that it is the very inclusion of these 'positive' elements that allows for a fuller understanding of human well-being (WHO 1947a, Larson 1996, Chang 2002). Intriguingly, however, while much has been made over the years of the inclusion of mental and social well-being, less attention has been accorded to the core of the definition – the absence of disease and infirmity. This is indeed an interesting lacuna, for although the definition does emphasize that health is not merely the absence of disease or infirmity, it is apparent that the absence of disease and infirmity are nevertheless considered the prerequisites for health. It therefore follows that the absence of disease and infirmity is central to the WHO's primary mission of securing the highest possible level of health for all peoples and, as such, it can be anticipated that the IO's secretariat would be expected to devote considerable attention to the eradication of disease in all its forms.

Further, investigation into the historical origins of the WHO also corroborates the heightened level of importance the organization was, and is, expected to assign to the task of preventing, controlling, and ideally eradicating epidemics. The 1946 International Health Conference that led to the creation of the WHO stipulated, for example, that every aspect of the IO's research and technical activities would 'have as their broad aim the more effective control and eventual eradication of disease' (WHO 1948b, p. 17). Likewise, in 1947, when discussing the delegated functions of the new universal health agency, the WHO Interim Commission concluded that 'the ultimate aim of the organisation must clearly be to wipe out the foci of these epidemics' (WHO 1947b, p. 14).

The epidemics that the Commission was referring to – cholera, plague, smallpox, yellow fever, and typhus – had already presented a considerable challenge to the international community in its attempts to control their spread. While it was never intended that the specific mention of these five diseases would preclude others, their devastating impact was recognized as requiring immediate action (Sawyer 1947), ultimately prompting their inclusion in the 1951 ISR.

Finally, aside from the WHO's explicit delegated obligation in Article 2 to work towards the eradication of infectious disease, three further provisions within the WHO Constitution underline the central importance of the organization's disease eradication responsibilities and the weight that the organization's founding members ascribed to this function. Under the first provision, located in Article 21, the WHA is authorized to adopt regulations relating to 'sanitary and quarantine requirements and other procedures designed to prevent the international spread of disease' (WHO 2005a, p. 7). This provision facilitated the creation of the ISR (later IHR), which, as previously discussed, form an integral part of the WHO's disease eradication delegation contract. The significance of this clause (and the importance the founders attached to the WHO's disease eradication function) is made further apparent, however, when taking note of the fact that unless member states explicitly request otherwise, every government must fully implement and adhere to any regulations or legislation passed by the WHA under this provision. The clause thus utilizes the principle known as 'contracting-out' (Burci and Vignes 2004, p. 132), and operates in direct contrast to the two-step process that member states traditionally follow when complying with international law: first by becoming a signatory, and then by formally ratifying the legislation through national legislative bodies.

The second provision, also contained within Article 21, permits the WHA to adopt 'nomenclatures with respect to diseases, causes of death and public health practices' (Article 21(b) – WHO 2005a, p. 7). This latter specification establishes the IO's information-gathering and categorization roles for all disease-related health complaints – a vital function that informs the allocation of resources and the development of appropriate measures aimed at preventing, containing, and eradicating disease. Indeed, without such data collection occurring, the international community would be largely oblivious to the number of, for example, cholera, HIV/AIDS, and cancer cases, and the resources required to treat them.

While both these provisions may initially appear inconsequential, they are in fact significant because they bestow upon the WHA the authority to exercise 'exceptional regulatory powers' which require only a two-thirds majority approval by member states to become automatically binding on all (Burci and Vignes 2004, p. 132). In effect, this means that even if a member state failed to endorse a new set of regulations passed by the WHA, the member state is required to either adhere to the new regulations or provide an explanation *and* obtain permission from the WHA for exemption (see WHO Constitution, Article 22). These exceptional powers thus attest to the considerable importance member states have attached to the WHO's function of preventing, controlling, and ideally eradicating infectious disease threats.

Third, and perhaps most significantly, a further provision located in Article 28 of the WHO Constitution authorizes the EB to confer upon the director-general emergency powers to respond to any event requiring 'immediate action'. Although a definition of what constitutes 'emergency powers' (or indeed even the extent of those powers) has never been explicitly outlined within the scope of either the Constitution or EB regulations, the emergence of epidemics is cited as one example where these powers may be conferred. Further, in the event that such powers are deemed necessary, the director-general is authorized to utilize every available resource at the organization's disposal to respond to the disaster. This provision is thereby notable for the exceptional power and autonomy it grants to the WHO's bureaucracy which, according to the terms of this clause, is not required to obtain the WHA's (i.e. member states') prior approval before enacting it. This third provision, which also forms part of the WHO's overall disease eradication contract with member states, thus provides one avenue where the IO's bureaucracy can exercise extensive power and authority that is ultimately only restricted by the organization's financial and technical resources. By endorsing Article 28, it can additionally be interpreted that member states consider the emergence of epidemics to be significant enough to warrant the temporary suspension of the organization's standard mechanisms of control.

Of course, at the same time it must be recalled that the founders of the WHO only ever intended for these exceptional powers to be activated for the benefit of member states. It is in this regard that the emphasis placed on the prevention, control, and eradication of infectious diseases is not entirely unexpected. The majority of the former International Sanitary Conferences of the 19th century were convened specifically in response to the threat from the 'Asian' diseases of cholera and plague (Briggs 1961). By the 20th century, the rise of germ theory, modern bacteriology, and specific medical treatments for individual diseases cemented the biomedical view of health as the dominant discourse, and with it, a focus on eliminating disease (Brandt and Gardner 2000). While the WHO's overt adoption of the concept of eradication was a new development (Goodman 1952, p. 74), the overall emphasis on disease prevention and control resonated strongly with the historical origins of international health collaboration more generally and in the 20th century specifically.

Moreover, assigning the IO to perform these tasks directly served the founding (and contemporary) member states' interests in at least two notable ways. Firstly, infectious disease outbreaks pose a direct threat to the social contract between governments and their citizens. Were disease outbreaks and epidemics allowed to rage unchecked, it was feared that the legitimacy of the state would be questioned for not offering sufficient protection to its citizens (Carrin 2006). Assigning this duty to an IO thereby alleviates some of the responsibility that individual administrations would otherwise have to assume. Secondly, the emphasis on diseases fits very comfortably within the biomedical model of health which, with its emphasis on objective measurement and verifiable facts, affords governments greater opportunity to measure the performance of the WHO – a critical factor for assessing whether the IO is adhering to its delegation contract as intended.

Indeed, it is important to recall that the WHO remains an intergovernmental organization answerable to its 194 member states. As sovereign entities, member states retain the authority over their respective territories and populations. They also may, at least theoretically and if sufficient numbers approve, revoke the organization's mandate and authority. This is the nature of the delegated authority (Sarooshi 2005). But it also places the WHO in an awkward, and at times unenviable, position whereby the WHO is accountable to member states for pursuing its delegated duties and yet may, whether by intention or omission, be prevented from doing so by those same member states if they are dissatisfied with the IO's behaviour or actions in any way. This situation therefore begs the question: What is the envisaged authority and autonomy of the WHO? Or, said another way, in what capacity is the WHO expected to fulfil its disease eradication delegation contract while interacting with sovereign member states?

In fact, in accordance with the very explicit vision enunciated by the WHO's founders, delegates at the 1946 International Health Conference determined the organization was 'to act as the directing and coordinating authority on international health work' (Article 2, WHO Constitution – WHO 2005a, p. 2). This overall mandate, which interestingly was moved to being cited as a function of the IO instead of it remaining as the central objective that all other functions were intended to guarantee (WHO 1947a, p. 70), is enshrined under Article 2 of the WHO Constitution and has been subsequently endorsed by every member state. Importantly however, it can be observed to embody two distinct forms of authority: *directing* and *coordinating*. The demarcation that can consequently be drawn is that the founders anticipated the organization would act in a controlling or supervisory capacity (directing), as well as acting as a unifying force, channelling the international community's efforts into a singular purpose (coordinating). When combined, these two forms of authority thus empower the WHO – at least in principle – to act as the lead technical agency in all international health matters.

In addition to the WHO's intended preeminent status, and arguably equally important for the WHO's health-for-security mandate, the framers of the new universal health organization also proposed that the WHO was to be endowed with 'a proper degree of autonomy' (WHO 1947a, p. 10). To facilitate this, specific features were deliberately incorporated into the IO's institutional design, such as conditions surrounding the appointment of staff, the organization's ability to set normative standards, and the regional office structure. It was also intended that the WHO would enjoy a measure of autonomy from its status as a specialized agency (Sharp 1947).

As noted earlier, the WHO's institutional design was broadly modelled on that of its parent organization, the UN. Yet while there are similarities in terms of internal composition to other IOs of the UN system (see Sands and Klein 2001, Gordenker 2005), it was also intended that each specialized agency should have unique characteristics. For instance, the World Bank Group is capable of generating at least 80 per cent of the revenue it requires to function through trading in private capital markets. Thus, unlike the majority of its counterparts that are beholden to member states for regular contributions and extrabudgetary funds (including the WHO), the World Bank is, to all intents and purposes, financially autonomous from its member states. When combined with other facets of the IO's institutional design, this grants the Bank's Board of Governors a measure of independence to determine the organization's policies (Nielson and Tierney 2003), as they are able to avoid one of the more compelling mechanisms of control that member states can exercise.

In a similar fashion, the International Civil Aviation Organization (ICAO) has a great deal more discretion in appointing the members of its organ of limited composition, the ICAO's Council. Unlike the WHO's EB, for example, which stipulates that there must be equal regional distribution in representation (Lerer and Matzopoulos 2001), the appointment of delegates to the ICAO's Council grants representation to the states most directly and immediately affected by the organization's activities (Sands and Klein 2001). Further, as no requirement exists to ensure equitable distribution of representation between regions, it is conceivable that the ICAO's Council, which has the authority to produce standards that all ICAO members must adhere to (Alvarez 2005), could, for instance, be comprised solely of European countries or a combination of North and South American countries. Hence, each specialized agency can have different characteristics in terms of operating procedures, decision-making processes, dispute resolution practices, the level and extent of IO autonomy, among several others (Schermers and Blokker 2003). Put simply another way, in line with Mitrany's Functional Theory of International Organization that suggested form should follow function (Mitrany 1945), each IO's institutional design should have distinct characteristics that reflect the nature of the work the IO was created to undertake (Beigbeder 1998).

It should not therefore be unexpected that several features of the WHO's institutional design reflect the IO's specific health focus. For instance, the Constitution identifies that delegates attending the WHA must 'be chosen from among persons most qualified by their technical competence in the field of health, preferably representing the national health administration of the member' (Article 11 – WHO 2005a, p. 5). Equivalent stipulations, which are intended to reflect the technical nature of the organization's work, also originally extended to the appointment of members to the EB. Moreover, aside from the compromise that was struck to incorporate the Americas' regional organization, as Burci and Vignes (2004, p. 17) identify, concerns regarding the technical nature of the WHO's work were a motivating factor in the decision not only to establish regional offices, but also to grant those offices a large measure of autonomy, as it was believed they 'would be more effective in solving local health problems'. Arguably, however, the greatest source of the WHO's autonomy was intended to be its administrative element, the secretariat.

The secretariat of any IO is, at its most basic, a large bureaucracy, often with its own internal culture and perspectives regarding the purpose and function of the institution (Barnett and Finnemore 2004). Partially substantiating Mitrany's treatise that allegiances are capable of shifting, it is not uncommon for the staff of IOs to develop loyalties to the institution they serve, fiercely protecting its interests and reputation. While it is accepted that this loyalty may be connected to some degree to ongoing job security (such as it is, given the extensiveness of short-term contracts), it is equally the case that many of the staff working for IOs have chosen to do so because of their belief in either the institution, its mandate, or a sense of moral obligation and/or public service. Moreover, as Barnett and Finnemore (ibid., p. 5) have observed, governments 'may actually want autonomous action from IO staff. Indeed, they often create an IO and invest it with considerable autonomy precisely because they are neither able nor willing to perform the IO's mission themselves'.

In the specific context of the WHO, it is quite clear that the founders of the organization intended for the secretariat to exercise considerable autonomy. For example, it was explicitly decreed:

> [T]he Director-General and the staff shall not seek or receive instructions from any government or from any authority external to the Organization. They shall refrain from any action which might reflect on their position as international officers. Each Member of the Organization on its part undertakes to respect the exclusively international character of the Director-General and the staff and not seek to influence them. (Article 37, WHO Constitution – WHO 2005a, p. 10)

Further, although the director-general is constitutionally required to give due regard 'to the importance of recruiting the staff on as wide a geographical basis as possible' (Article 35 – ibid.), considerable weight is also placed on the technical expertise and staff qualifications (see Article 30), so much so that the WHO has at times been described as consisting of the 'medical mafia' (Elling 1981, p. 42). To avoid any notion that these stipulations are a relic of a former era though, it is also worth highlighting that by periodically affirming the IO's staff regulations – which is constitutionally required under Article 35 – member states have repeatedly encouraged the secretariat to act exclusively in the interests of the WHO, eschewing subjugation to any 'external authority' (section 1.10 of Staff Regulations of the WHO).[3] These various stipulations speak to the quintessential nature of the WHO's intended autonomy and the extent to which member states recognize the benefit of (limited) independence.

Thus, not only is it evident that the founding member states anticipated that the WHO would serve as the directing and coordinating authority in all international health matters, it is also apparent that they expected the organization's bureaucracy would exercise considerable discretion as an impartial, autonomous IO while pursuing its overall mission. As one commentator went on to observe at the time:

> Clearly it is the intent of all these provisions that WHO shall function as one of the "planets" in the "solar" system of the United Nations. Even so, the founders of the Organization gave emphatic expression to their conviction that it must retain substantial operational autonomy. This point of view was notably reflected in the name they selected for the new institution, in the position they took as to the location of its permanent seat, and in the character of the agreement they had in mind for its affiliation with the UN. (Sharp 1947, p. 528)

Crucially, however, this is not to suggest that the WHO's autonomy and authority was ever intended to be absolute. In fact, the organization's founding member states were keen to ensure that several mechanisms of control were designed into the WHO's institutional structure in order to prevent illicit IO behaviour or mission creep emerging. The following brief section will discuss these limitations and constraints on the WHO's authority and autonomy, prior to examining three of the WHO's disease eradication programmes for malaria, smallpox, and TB in the next chapter.

The limits of the WHO's authority and autonomy

As noted above, the WHO is an intergovernmental organization. What this means in practice is that while the WHO has been authorized to act as the directing and coordinating authority in all international health matters and its bureaucracy has been granted considerable autonomy to determine the most appropriate means of fulfilling the IO's primary mission, the organization nevertheless remains accountable to its member states or principals. In order to ensure that accountability continues, member states have also built several mechanisms of control into the organization's institutional design by inserting various provisions or qualifications into the WHO's constitutive treaty (i.e. the WHO Constitution). These mechanisms, which may be broadly categorized as politico-legal and economic, have in turn generated various technical and socio-legal constraints that ultimately serve to limit the IO's authority and autonomy, and are thereby intended to prevent unplanned behaviour or transaction costs from arising.

In terms of the WHO's politico-legal constraints, the first and most significant can be found in Article 2 of the WHO Constitution. Article 2(c) states unambiguously that the WHO is 'to assist Governments, upon request, in strengthening health services' (WHO 2005a, p. 2). Likewise, Article 2(d) states that the WHO is 'to furnish appropriate technical assistance and, in emergencies, necessary aid upon the request or acceptance of Governments' (ibid.). When viewed in collaboration with the organization's delegated authority, it is thus apparent that although the founders of the WHO clearly intended for the organization to act as the directing and coordinating authority in all international health work, they did not intend for that authority to extend to infringing the sovereignty of its member states. As Beigbeder (1998, p. 15) has succinctly noted, the WHO's authority 'cannot be imposed upon Member States'. Rather, reflecting the conventional PA model of delegation, the organization was designed to be subservient, supporting member states only if and when they required assistance. These two provisions, prominent as they are in the Constitution, thereby firmly attest to the fact that the authority and autonomy of the WHO is not unqualified nor that it was ever intended to be.

Furthermore, the notion of a compliant but inoffensive IO has also been emphasized in several other clauses cited throughout the WHO Constitution. Under Article 18(a), for instance, the WHA maintains the power 'to determine the policies of the Organization' (WHO 2005a, p. 6). The WHA, which is comprised solely of member states, thereby possesses the final approval on what the organization's secretariat undertakes on their behalf and what it does not. Likewise, in accordance with Article 24 of the WHO Constitution, the WHA has the power to appoint and remove those members of the EB who are charged with executing the policies of the organization, or more precisely of the WHA. By configuring these features into the WHO's institutional design in this way, member states have clearly hoped to retain firm control and oversight over the IO, defining both its sphere of competence and preventing the organization's bureaucracy from exercising unrestrained authority and autonomy.

Not content with politico-legal constraints alone, however, the WHO's founding member states also insisted on a variety of control mechanisms designed to restrain the IO's authority and autonomy through economic means. Specifically, as articulated in Article 18(f), the founders ensured that member states in the form of the WHA retained the right 'to supervise the financial policies of the Organization and to review and approve the budget' (ibid.). This authority, which has been further endorsed and expanded in Article 56 of the Constitution, thus delimits in a very pragmatic way what the organization may and may not accomplish. By inserting these provisions it may be correspondingly interpreted that, with the exception of health emergencies requiring immediate action, the founders sought to thwart unmitigated bureaucratic autonomy being exercised by the WHO's secretariat and director-general. In addition, such oversight procedures also allow member states to limit, if they so choose, the WHO's ability to act as the directing and coordinating authority in *all* international health matters, and by default curtail the organization's overall authority.

Of course, in practice the politico-legal and economic constraints have also combined to generate a variety of secondary controls on the authority and autonomy of the WHO. These have perhaps been most keenly felt in relation to the organization's technical prowess. Since the 1980s, the WHO's budget has remained tightly constrained due to member states' continued insistence on zero-growth of the UN specialized agencies' budgets (Vaughan et al. 1995). Indeed, despite the IO's global health mandate, in 2001 its budget was estimated as equivalent to approximately two and a half hours of global military expenditure (Benatar 2001). Not surprisingly, this situation has not been improved in the wake of the 2008 financial crisis. As Burci and Vignes (2004, p. 195) have observed, the outcome of these policies has been that 'WHO's technical cooperation mainly consists of advisory services rather than financial aid or operational activities'. The associated paradox has been that while politically it remains accountable to member states for achieving its mission, operationally the WHO has persistently lacked the material means to do so.

The logical conclusion to be drawn is that the WHO's member states are very aware of the effects that placing such limitations on the organization's capabilities engender. The extent of the WHO's authority and autonomy has thus potentially been best captured by Sharp (1947, p. 520) when he states:

> In realistic terms it may be said that WHO will be able to move toward its central objective only insofar as it can prod governments and private groups to provide services and initiate programmes they might not otherwise undertake. The financial and technical resources essential to its work will be forthcoming only in the degree that Member states, chiefly a few of the richer ones, are willing to supply them. During the earlier phases of its life the new Organization will probably not have either the means or the authority to conduct extensive field activities comparable to those of an advanced national health administration though such developments may come later. The role of WHO will be primarily that of a catalytic agent.

Given this state of affairs, it is perhaps not surprising that the WHO secretariat (including the director-general) have come to rely very heavily upon the organization's normative power and reputation (socio-legal status) to effect influence. In fact, as the founders envisaged, in many ways it is the WHO's ability to act as an impartial, independent organization in possession of consummate health expertise that is the WHO's greatest resource. As a consequence, the WHO bureaucracy has become very protective of its reputation as an objective, efficient, and effective IO (Burci and Vignes 2004, p. 99). At the same time, it is equally important to note that even when the organization has met these conditions, the WHO's reputation alone has not automatically resulted in member states' adjusting their policies. One contemporary example highlighting this reality, which also directly relates to the WHO's now-global health security mandate, transpired in 2003, when Nigeria refused to fully participate in the Global Polio Eradication Initiative (GPEI) (Raufu 2004a).

The WHO initiated the GPEI programme in 1988 in collaboration with three partner organizations, with the stated objective of eradicating poliomyelitis worldwide by the year 2005 (GPEI 2013). Although the Nigerian government initially participated in the global programme, four areas within Nigeria suspended vaccination initiatives in mid-October 2003, expressing fears that the programme was part of a US plot to depopulate Muslim territories by causing sterility and spreading HIV/AIDS (Fleck 2004, Raufu 2004b). By September 2004 polio cases had again begun to reappear in large numbers throughout Nigeria, spreading to surrounding countries. Nigeria's refusal to fully participate thereby threatened the GPEI's success and was potentially exposing the world's population to a global resurgence of a debilitating and oftentimes fatal disease (Heymann and Aylward 2004). Yet despite this development, the only option available to the WHO was to utilize its partner organizations, neighbouring governments, and international media sources in an attempt to pressure those non-compliant areas into re-commencing their vaccination initiatives (Schlein 2003). As a consequence, Nigeria did resume its polio eradication programme in late 2004, but not before an extensive epidemic was initiated that has continued to set the ultimate goal of global eradication back years.

A similar situation then arose in Pakistan in 2012, following the decision of a local faction of the Taliban to boycott the GPEI programme underway in Waziristan in the Federally Administered Tribal Areas, Pakistan. Distrust of immunization programmes had been growing in the area since 2011, when it was revealed that the US Central Intelligence Agency had employed a local doctor to simulate a hepatitis vaccination programme as part of the efforts to track down Osama bin Laden (Mohammadi 2012). In late 2012, the Taliban's opposition took a more sinister turn when, tragically, some five local healthcare workers (HCW) engaged in the GPEI were murdered (Boseley 2012). As a result of these and continuing attacks, the programme has continued to experience periodic disruptions (WHO 2014b); these disruptions, while completely understandable and appropriate, have nevertheless served to hamper global eradication efforts.

A further example illustrating the limited technical and socio-legal abilities of the WHO that also directly impacts upon the organization's disease eradication function relates to its efforts to reduce global poverty. The correlations between poverty and communicable disease emergence are evident, multiple, and oftentimes mutually reinforcing. For instance, impoverished communities habitually lack access to many basic services such as clean water and sanitation. These factors, which tend to be compounded by chronic malnutrition, living in over-crowded and unhygienic surroundings, and inadequate ventilation and heating, contribute to conditions in which infectious diseases flourish. Moreover, as the Commission on Macroeconomics and Health (2001, p. 43) concluded, 'the poor may lack the knowledge to protect themselves adequately or seek the needed services; they may lack the power to protect their rights; or they may lack income to access services'. Ultimately this dynamic generates a vicious cycle in which poverty leads to ill health (and specifically, exposure to infectious diseases), which in turn often leads to further poverty.

The WHO's bureaucracy long ago recognized the parallels between poverty and disease emergence, yet it was only after 1998 that the IO began to explicitly explore and participate in addressing poverty-related issues (WHO 1999a). The important caveat to the WHO's efforts in this area is, however, that the organization remains strictly relegated to a consultative role. While this is in part understandable given that the WHO's focus is not poverty reduction per se, by retaining tight control of the IO's budget, member states have nevertheless used their control oversight mechanisms to great effect, preventing the WHO's bureaucracy from independently expanding its field of activity. As a result, the WHO secretariat internalized the sentiment that any further expansion of the organization's role in this area is not considered appropriate or feasible (Burci and Vignes 2004). Rather, it has chosen to highlight the inequalities and the lack of investment in healthcare services in an attempt to encourage (and embarrass) member states into allocating more resources to address 'the causes of the causes' of ill health (Horton 2002) – measures that, as the lack of progress in achieving the Millennium Development Goals (MDGs) attests to, have met with mixed success (Tan et al. 2003, Ruxin et al. 2005).

Conclusion

In summary, it is evident that the WHO has an incontestable mandate for ensuring international security via the elimination of infectious diseases. Not only was the elimination of infectious diseases explicitly outlined in the WHO's Constitution when the organization was founded, the passage of subsequent framework agreements (such as the IHR 2005 and 2011 PIP Framework) and multiple WHA resolutions have formed an implicit disease eradication delegation contract with the IO's member states. This 'health-for-security' contract is also reflected to an extent in the WHO's own definition of health, which while emphasizing social and mental well-being, identifies the absence of disease and infirmity as the minimum benchmark for human health. The WHO secretariat therefore has both a moral and legal obligation to assist member states in preventing, controlling, and eliminating infectious diseases wherever and whenever such diseases arise. To facilitate this work, the founders of the organization empowered the WHO to serve as the directing and coordinating authority in international health, imbuing the organization's bureaucracy with considerable authority and autonomy.

Still, as exemplified by the questions that arose regarding the WHO's management of the 2003 SARS outbreak and the 2009 H1N1 influenza pandemic (which are explored in greater depth in subsequent chapters), that authority is not absolute. Nor, as this chapter has discussed, was that authority ever intended to be. For despite the authority and autonomy that the organization was granted, the founders of the WHO also ensured that several mechanisms of control were integrated into the WHO's institutional design. This was done in order to avoid illicit IO behaviour arising, to protect member states' sovereignty, and to ensure that member states continued to retain broad oversight and control of the WHO. These mechanisms – which include several politico-legal and economic controls that have in turn generated further constraints of a technical and socio-legal nature – reaffirm the subservient nature of the IO to its member states and constrain the WHO secretariat's powers.

2
The WHO's Classical Approach to Disease Eradication

Virtually upon its creation, and at the urging of the organization's member states, the WHO secretariat immediately set about exercising its newly bestowed powers in disease prevention, control, and eradication. This chapter explores three of the WHO's disease eradication initiatives – the MEP, the SEP, and the WHO's attempts to eliminate tuberculosis (Global TB Programme). Drawing on Haas' typology of IO learning (1990, pp. 17–49), attention will be given to identifying where there is evidence of epistemic communities having formed alliances with key partners to advance their own agenda. In addition, the chapter identifies and compares the roles that the WHO secretariat assumed throughout the eradication campaigns, as well as the organization's overall governance approach. In so doing, it is apparent that there is evidence to suggest that the IO learned from past mistakes and developed a standard or classical approach to managing infectious disease threats – an approach which, as will be discussed in the next chapter, was then radically reshaped around the time of the 2003 SARS outbreak.

These three campaigns – the MEP, SEP, and the Global TB Programme – were selected principally because they represent some of the WHO secretariat's first attempts at fulfilling the IO's health-for-security mandate. The MEP, for instance, was the first global campaign ever launched to eradicate a disease, and yet it proved a monumental failure. In contrast, the SEP, which was launched even as the failures of the MEP were becoming apparent, is hailed to this day as the WHO's greatest success. Like the MEP, the WHO's programme to eradicate TB also proved unsuccessful, resulting in the bureaucracy downgrading its objective from eradication to disease control, exemplified by the current (and ongoing) Stop TB campaign. Nonetheless, despite the three initiatives' varying levels of success, a clear management style emerged – one in which the WHO secretariat can be seen to perform particular roles and functions while eschewing its constitutional authority to direct international health work, preferring instead to adopt a more circumspect approach of facilitating cooperation wherever it was (and is) more politically feasible.

The Malaria Eradication Programme

The world's first-ever truly global attempt at eradicating a communicable disease was officially launched by the Eighth WHA in 1955 with the adoption of resolution *WHA8.30 Malaria eradication*. With this one act, governments around the world committed both themselves and the WHO to an unprecedented public health initiative: the elimination of all forms of human malaria.[1] The resolution, which encouraged all governments to intensify their efforts before *anopheline* mosquito resistance to insecticides became widespread, authorized the director-general to undertake measures aimed at persuading those governments not already pursuing malaria eradication to do so. The resolution also allowed for the creation of a new special account to finance the eradication programme, and under the terms of the resolution the director-general was permitted to solicit funds from both governments and private sector contributors for the purpose of financing the initiative. Most significantly, the resolution required that the WHO amend its policy of malaria control to that of eradication – a policy that ultimately proved disastrous for the IO's reputation. In fact, given that the failure of the MEP has often been attributed to the WHO's mismanagement, it is significant that the secretariat had initially advocated a policy of malaria control, only amending it to eradication when member states insisted in 1955 that the policy be changed.

By 1946 malaria epidemics had become a frequent, even yearly, occurrence in many parts of the world. Those countries ravaged by WWI were particularly adversely affected, and with the outbreak of hostilities in 1939 further disrupting the supply of anti-malarial drugs and causing extensive damage to healthcare infrastructure and medical services, the situation rapidly worsened (Goodman 1952, p. 142, Humphreys 1996). At the same time however, technological developments throughout WWII – particularly in the form of dichloro-diphenyl-trichloroethane (DDT) – appeared to offer for the first time the distinct possibility that malaria may actually be eradicable. As a result, the Interim Commission of the WHO determined that 'special attention' should be accorded to controlling the disease (WHO 1948a, p. 31), and in 1947 the Commission established the Expert Committee on Malaria to determine the organization's policy on the matter.

Based on the Expert Committee's recommendations, the WHO secretariat subsequently instigated a limited technical assistance programme of malaria control as early as May 1948. The position adopted by the organization was therefore significant in that it contrasted with a small, albeit growing number of prominent public health practitioners who advocated that malaria eradication should be pursued through the widespread use of DDT residual spraying and orally administered medications such as chloroquine. Instead, the Expert Committee had urged that the IO should adopt policies and procedures that utilized a variety of control methods and techniques. Moreover, rather than envisaging an aggressive role for the WHO, the Committee recommended that the organization's bureaucracy limit itself to that of evaluating existing control measures, providing expert advice, conducting disease surveillance, and promoting 'the production of insecticides and therapeutic agents and improvement of their distribution' (WHO 1948d, p. 5). Where necessary and upon request, 'demonstration teams' of medical personnel would also instruct national health authorities in the best disease control practices (Siddiqi 1995, pp. 128–130). The role proposed by the Expert Committee for the WHO was thus nominal, providing technical assistance only where required while advancing a policy of disease control.

Nevertheless, by 1955 it had become clear that the WHO's stance towards malaria eradication was untenable. Somewhat ironically, according to contemporary standards the WHO's initial policy of malaria control would be viewed as rational and measured, but by the mid-1950s the IO's policy was viewed as redundant and incongruent with the scientific consensus of the time. A number of campaigns to eradicate malaria were already underway, headed by such organizations as the Rockefeller Foundation, the UNRRA, the UN International Children's Emergency Fund (UNICEF), and the PASB. Moreover, in contrast to the WHO's policy the other IOs were utilizing DDT residual spraying as their central strategy and were observing 'spectacular results' (WHO 1947b, pp. 182–184). Intriguingly, the fact that resistance to DDT was appearing failed to dissuade the medical establishment (Calder 1958), instead spurring them to advocate even more vehemently that eradication could be achieved if – and only if – action was taken immediately. The WHO was subsequently deemed to be the most appropriate vehicle for achieving such action. Sensing that considerable international momentum had built, little resistance was offered by the WHO secretariat when it was proposed that the IO should amend its control strategy to that of eradication.

Following the adoption of resolution WHA8.30, both the WHO's existing policy and activities underwent some notable changes. The most apparent and immediate effect was that the policy of malaria control was expunged as the WHO's senior executives – many of whom were malariologists who had by the mid-1950s been advocating eradication for years (including, notably, the director-general)[2] – shifted the organization's focus to pursuing the elimination of all forms of human malaria. Turning to the WHO Expert Committee on Malaria for guidance, the methodology the WHO proposed for achieving this goal consisted of four clearly defined phases: preparatory, attack, consolidation, and maintenance (WHO 1956a, pp. 3–4); and at the urging of the IO, every national campaign was subsequently modelled on this one design (Gramiccia and Beales 1988, p. 1349, Bruce-Chwatt 1998, p. 50).

Significantly, the WHO additionally advocated that the global eradication could be realistically achieved within one decade so long as each country adhered to the recommended timeframes and protocols (WHO 1955, p. 199, Siddiqi 1995, p. 165). For those countries that lacked their own expertise the WHO then issued a series of highly prescriptive, very detailed protocols produced by the Expert Committee on Malaria that covered such topics as the type of compressors to be used in spraying; the amount of insecticide required per square metre; even the structure and number of personnel required for DDT spraying squads. Every country undertaking an eradication programme was advised to incorporate these protocols into their respective campaign, and WHO consultants were made available to assist each national health authority to comply.

By 1958 some 63 countries had either commenced new campaigns or converted their former malaria control programmes to pursue eradication (Yekutiel 1981, p. 469). Demand for WHO guidance and technical assistance grew rapidly as a result, prompting the organization to virtually double its MEP-dedicated staff in the first 10 years of the programme's operation. Particular emphasis was placed on the speed and efficiency of reporting and, in contrast to the secretariat's usual tendency to rely on national health authorities to report cases and/or outbreaks at their own discretion, the WHO provided its own staff to assist in the collection of data. At the WHO headquarters in Geneva, the secretariat also intensified its role as a sorting house for epidemic intelligence data, disseminating this information as fast as possible to assist in the planning and implementation of eradication campaigns. In the field, WHO personnel worked with national health authorities to apply the organization's policies with military-style precision, ensuring that – as much as possible – each country's eradication programme adhered to the model, timeframe, and recommendations of the secretariat (Cochi et al. 1998).

It is in this regard that the WHO was observed to adapt a highly structured approach to malaria eradication and, at least initially, the global campaign appeared to validate this rigid, command-and-control approach. Seeking to attest to the programme's usefulness, the WHO was observed to claim as early as March 1957 that at least 10 countries had already either 'practically or totally' achieved eradication (WHO 1957a, p. 533). While this was later proved to be premature, by 1967 the WHO had certified 13 countries as having completely eradicated malaria (WHO 1968a, p. 165), and by 1968 it had been estimated that some 997 million people living in previously malaria-endemic regions had been freed from the risk of transmission (WHO 1969a, p. 109). In fact, even in spite of the later criticisms, the programme did achieve amazing results and was a remarkable accomplishment. As Beales and Gilles (2002, p. 111) observe:

> The achievements of the WHO Malaria Eradication Campaign were quite remarkable at a time when no form of health services whatsoever penetrated into most endemic villages and there were no roads, bridges, railway lines, airports, electricity or telephones and, therefore, very limited population movements. Much of the work was carried out on foot, by boat, by donkey, horse or camel back where vehicles could not penetrate. Millions of people were freed from the burden of this disease and large areas of land were opened up to agriculture and industrial development because of it.

Despite these notable achievements, however, in the end the WHO failed in its attempt to eliminate all forms of human malaria, and the MEP was officially suspended in 1973. The closure of the MEP combined with the recognition that it had fallen short of its target, not surprisingly, reflected poorly on the WHO as the organization charged with ensuring the programme's success. Moreover, many of these criticisms were not without cause. As can be observed from even the brief summary provided above, while in one sense the IO may be assumed to have acted as envisaged – fulfilling its role as the directing and coordinating authority in international health – at the same time, the inflexible, authoritarian style of governance employed by the WHO bureaucracy arguably contributed to the programme's failure.

For example, one of the first recognizable limitations of the MEP was the evident lack of planning prior to the programme's rollout. As noted above, it had been initially suggested by the WHO in 1955 that global eradication could be achieved within 10 years of the programme's commencement. Each individual national campaign was subsequently designed according to this timeframe, and the various financial contributors co-opted into the global campaign were assured that their support would only be required for a correspondingly brief period (see, for example, Black 1986, Siddiqi 1995). Operational, logistical, and technical difficulties soon demolished the projected target date, however; and given that little scope within the planning stage had been granted for extensions, contributors and supporters of the programme understandably became disillusioned when the targets were not achieved. One of the consequences of this disillusionment was that the major donors, namely UNICEF and the government of the United States, began to impose harsher criteria under which their funding would be provided (Black 1986). As evidence increasingly began to emerge in the late 1960s that the original target date was not going to be achieved, and that even the goal of eradication might prove elusive, both major donors completely withdrew their financial support.

Inflated, unrealistic expectations also contributed to a level of disillusionment amongst member states involved in the programme. This was observed to have a direct negative impact upon a limited number of national campaigns, particularly when operational and technical difficulties such as mosquito resistance and external aid shortages were encountered that had not been adequately planned for (WHO 1960a, 1967a). In many developing countries, already lacking sufficient infrastructure to support a prolonged eradication campaign, some of these impediments proved too costly, resulting in their abandoning the global programme in all but name (WHO 1965a, Gupte et al. 2001, Tren and Bate 2001). Such outcomes further complicated the WHO's efforts to shore-up ongoing support for the programme as the anticipated declarations of complete eradication consequently fell short of the campaign's earlier achievements.

Yet a further complication of the WHO's governance of the MEP, and one which certainly contributed to the programme's ultimate demise, was the lack of autonomy granted to individual national campaigns. As noted above, under the terms established by the WHO, each local programme was to adopt the four-phase method for malaria eradication that relied overwhelmingly on the DDT residual spraying technique.[3] According to this strategy, which was overseen by the organization and linked to the provision of funding and resources, each local campaign was required to focus primarily on eradicating the vector of malaria transmission by spraying every household with DDT. Significantly though, the WHO's policy completely ignored 'non-human' dwellings such as stables and barns, under the mistaken belief that malaria-carrying mosquitoes would not reside there (Gramiccia and Beales 1988, p. 1353). The corollary of this decision was that a key vector habitat was left untreated, raising the likelihood that re-infestation of human dwellings would occur. While this was just one example, various other problems relating to the lack of local authorities' autonomy to amend this strategy soon manifested themselves as well.

For instance, one of the first difficulties to emerge as a direct result of the inability to adapt the central strategy of DDT spraying was the challenge presented by insecticide resistance. Provoked by the programme's over-reliance on the one chemical, by 1968 it was noted that some 56 species of mosquitoes had developed resistance specifically to DDT (WHO 1970). The end result of this development was that the global campaign's achievements were gradually, steadily reversed. Yet because local campaigns were actively discouraged from either amending or employing other proven control methods such as the application of alternative insecticides or the supply of anti-malarial medications (WHO 1956a, Bruce-Chwatt 1998), the WHO's decision to retain central administrative oversight of local campaigns paradoxically undermined the very effectiveness of the global programme itself.

Problems arising from the lack of local autonomy in being able to amend the strategy of residual spraying also manifested in other ways as well. Specifically, in countries that possessed a high proportion of nomadic population groups, many of whom possessed no permanent dwellings, either sleeping in the open or in semi-permanent structures that were not fully enclosed, the strategy of residual spraying was often rendered useless (WHO 1960c, pp. 1–4). In other countries such as Thailand, Laos, and Vietnam, whose populations lived in mountainous regions and very humid climates, walled structures were not commonly found, making the central strategy of the MEP almost entirely redundant (Gramiccia and Beales 1988). Added to this were general concerns regarding the environmental impact of widespread DDT spraying, particularly on flora and fauna (Stapleton 2004). Yet despite these considerations, often there was very little provision for local authorities to amend their respective campaigns to meet local conditions, resulting in the corresponding outcome that the MEP was not achieving the results that had been promised.

It is also pertinent to note at this juncture that the inflexibility regarding the central strategy of DDT residual spraying arose, at least in part, from an earlier decision of the WHO bureaucracy not to undertake research into developing new malaria eradication techniques. This evasion of the IO's constitutionally mandated obligation notably occurred at the commencement of the programme, as it was naively believed at the time that existing technologies were sufficient to achieve global eradication. This belief, based on the Expert Committee on Malaria's recommendations, allowed the WHO's senior leadership to adamantly maintain that global eradication could be achieved through the rigid application of DDT and the oral administration of chloroquine alone. As such, granting local campaigns the ability to deviate from this policy was perceived to threaten the success of the overall programme and should not, therefore, be permitted (Fenner et al. 1988). In the end, the WHO's decision to avoid undertaking further research on malaria eradication techniques contributed to the overall collapse of the programme.

Finally, one of the foremost operational limitations of the programme, and of the organization that correspondingly administered it, was the complete exclusion of large malaria-endemic regions. Indeed, two groups of countries were purposely debarred with the full consent and knowledge of the WHO – the first reportedly on technical grounds and the second on the basis of political considerations. The first group of countries, located in sub-Saharan Africa, were excluded on the basis that malaria was assumed to be far too endemic, and that the countries were far too underdeveloped for the programme to even be attempted (WHO 1957b). This decision, which was entirely antithetical to the concept of global eradication, thereby left the region that suffered the highest prevalence of malaria completely untouched. The second group of countries, consisting of the People's Republic of China, North Korea, and North Vietnam, were largely excluded on the grounds of their status as nonmember states. While their exclusion reflected equally on the governments of these countries – each of whom had declined to join the WHO and the global effort for their own political reasons – little attempt was made to encourage their inclusion. The corollary of this development was that even if the programme had succeeded in every other region of the world, their continued exclusion would have undermined the global campaign's overall objective of complete eradication and raised the prospect of re-infestation once the attack phase of the MEP had been completed.

From the above exegesis it can thus be surmised that the WHO adopted a very particular style of governance throughout the duration of the MEP.

The IO not only functioned as the international community's directing and coordinating authority, it also performed three very distinct roles: that of epidemic intelligence consolidator, policy prescriber, and government assessor. In the first instance, for example, rather than encouraging that new research should be conducted into improving eradication techniques, the organization's bureaucracy, assuming that it had obtained sufficient understanding of how to achieve global eradication, consolidated the scientific community's existing knowledge into very prescriptive, detailed instructions for implementation. On the basis of the medical advice provided at the time, the WHO bureaucracy assumed that alternative options were irrelevant and that new research was unwarranted. Further, and explicitly related to the above, although the WHO did recognize the importance of disease surveillance and continued to collect, analyze, and disseminate the information it received, the IO's bureaucracy failed to utilize this information to consider the impact of its own policies. The WHO thus simply consolidated the epidemic intelligence it obtained, passively and uncritically accepting that the programme's overall lack of progress (and eventual failure) was attributable to poor execution by member states.

Surprisingly, and in spite of the above, the WHO also assumed the role of policy prescriber, dictating to countries what, when, where, and how they were to construct their respective eradication campaigns. Of course, as outlined above, it has to be acknowledged that the WHO did not generate the initial policy of malaria eradication – this was instigated by member states in a classic example of principal delegation. Nonetheless, once the IO was empowered to commence the global programme, it made full use of its constitutional authority. Intriguingly, the organization's bureaucracy accomplished this feat even though all reference to the WHO's directing authority had been purposefully removed from the 1955 WHA resolution, reportedly in respect to member states' sovereignty (WHO 1955, pp. 230–232, 239). Whether this development then derived from the fact that an eradication campaign of this magnitude had never previously been attempted, or from some misguided perception on behalf of member states that the recently created health agency possessed some previously unforeseen extraordinary competence, is unclear. The reality that nevertheless emerged was that governments the world over acquiesced to the WHO's authority, in many instances unswervingly adhering to its policies. Throughout the duration of the MEP, the WHO thus served as the international community's directing and coordinating authority, as originally envisaged by the founders. Yet the failure of the programme equally harmed the reputation of the organization, its bureaucracy, and, as will be discussed further below, the WHO's attempts to undertake future global disease eradication campaigns.

Third, whether or not it emerged as an unintentional by-product of the WHO's methods, the organization's bureaucracy also effectively served as government assessor for a number of countries participating in the MEP. This was most clearly demonstrated when some of the programme's major donors threatened to withhold funding from those countries not adhering to WHO policies. Although not instigated by the organization itself, the bureaucracy nevertheless failed to intervene, thereby tacitly signalling their endorsement of the policy. The WHO's role as government assessor was also demonstrated by the IO's refusal to include certain geographical regions within the global campaign on the basis of technical and political grounds. In each of these circumstances the organization's bureaucracy, to all intents and purposes, acted as an assessor of member states, determining which countries were suitable candidates to receive assistance in eradicating malaria and which were not.

Ultimately, when combined, all three roles did enable the organization to then assume the position of lead technical agency. However, the WHO responded to this global challenge in an authoritarian, almost dictatorial manner, requiring member states to adhere to its policies or face the possibility that they would be viewed as international pariahs unwilling to assist in the elimination of one of the world's most debilitating diseases. The failure of the programme – as the IO's first major initiative – understandably (and perhaps appropriately) resulted in raising serious concerns about the utility and benefit of the new universal health agency. The MEP thus had a significant impact upon the organization, both internally as the bureaucracy faced the reality that it had failed to achieve the goal of eliminating all forms of human malaria, and externally amongst member states dissatisfied with the IO's performance and competence.

The Smallpox Eradication Programme

The SEP remains to this day the WHO's – and quite possibly, the international community's – greatest achievement. The programme itself was executed in two distinct stages, and within 11 years of the intensified phase of the programme commencing, the last recorded case of human-to-human transmission occurred on 26 October 1977. Some three years later, after suitable time had elapsed to ensure no further transmissions transpired, the world was declared free of smallpox by the 33rd WHA on

8 May 1980. The WHA's declaration was momentous, signalling not only the successful completion of an international effort to eradicate a highly contagious, life-threatening disease, but also that more than 3,000 years of human suffering from smallpox had now finally come to an end.

It is therefore somewhat ironic, given that the SEP was so successful, that the global campaign suffered from a pervasive lack of interest from its foundation. In fact, although the triumph of the programme has been frequently attributed to the organization's leadership (see, for example, Henderson 1987a, Pratt 1999), it is interesting to note that with the exception of the WHO's first director-general, Dr Brock Chisholm, the IO's senior bureaucracy were extremely hesitant, even averse, to the suggestion of launching a smallpox eradication campaign. Further, in direct contrast to the MEP, the WHO's bureaucracy persistently displayed an unwillingness to provide global leadership on the matter, and this reticence continued even well into the intensified and final stage of the programme as the prospect of eradication was imminent.

The notion of launching a global campaign to eradicate smallpox was, intriguingly, first tabled at the Sixth WHA in 1953 by the then outgoing director-general, Dr Brock Chisholm. Seeking to build on the PASB's 1950 declaration to eliminate smallpox from the Americas, Dr Chisholm proposed that a global campaign would be a suitable endeavour for the newborn organization to pursue and that smallpox was an appropriate candidate for eradication. The proposal was rejected despite its support by highly influential public health figures such as Fred Soper (Kerr 1970, Fenner et al. 1988). The reasons cited by delegates at the WHA included that smallpox was considered by many countries to be a regional and local health problem rather than a disease requiring a global solution. Moreover, it was felt that the cost of a global campaign would be prohibitive. Thus even two years later as the global campaign to eradicate malaria was officially launched, the WHA simply advocated that 'health administrations conduct, wherever necessary, campaigns against smallpox as an integral part of their public-health programs' (WHO 1973, p. 90). To be sure, the vast majority of member states demonstrated so little interest that the suggestion of a global campaign to eradicate smallpox was correspondingly 'quietly buried' by the WHO bureaucracy for four years (Fenner et al. 1988, p. 392).

In 1959, some four years after the MEP had commenced, the WHA's position on smallpox eradication was reversed. Somewhat paradoxically, the WHA's about turn came at the insistence of the Union of Soviet Socialist Republics (USSR), which had only recently re-engaged with the organization after a brief period of estrangement. In an official report to the 11th WHA, the USSR's deputy health minister, Dr Viktor Zhdanov, urged the WHA to reconsider its former position, advocating that the complete eradication of smallpox could realistically be achieved within 10 years. Demonstrating its commitment to this objective, the USSR donated 25 million doses of the smallpox vaccine to the WHO to distribute as necessary (WHO 1959a), and sent various offers of assistance to countries throughout Asia and Western Africa where smallpox was known to be endemic (Fenner et al. 1988). Broadly endorsed by the majority of delegates, the WHA subsequently requested the new director-general, Dr Marcolino Candau, to prepare a report on the viability of a sustained global eradication campaign. The 12th WHA then approved the report and the director-general's proposals the following year (in spite of the serious misgivings of a number of member states), thereby launching the first stage of the organization's new worldwide strategy to eradicate the smallpox virus (Henderson 1977).

The initial SEP strategy developed by the WHO in the early 1960s was relatively straightforward: to vaccinate at least 80 per cent of all populations living in endemic countries, thus breaking the chain of transmission (WHO 1968c). Yet in direct contrast to the MEP, which by this time was operating at full capacity, in an evident case of IO shirking the WHO refused to provide detailed oversight of the programme, insisting instead that each individual country was to be entirely responsible for its own campaign's administration, execution, and expenses. The WHO maintained this position despite requests to the contrary from a number of its member states, stating that it would only provide technical assistance in the form of supplying vaccines (which were to be donated by member states and quality-tested by the WHO) and disease surveillance. If requested, one of the programme's five consultants could also be made available to advise on local implementation (Fenner et al. 1988). Not surprisingly, little progress was made; even in 1961, when several delegates of the WHA explicitly requested that the WHO redouble its efforts and establish 'a well-defined global eradication programme like the programme that existed in the case of malaria' (WHO 1962, pp. 284–286), the director-general actively sought to discourage the idea. Incredibly, this detached oversight of the initial phase of the SEP continued for at least the first five years of the programme's operation, much to the sustained frustration of the USSR and other member states who repeatedly called for greater involvement from the IO in generating support for and managing the SEP.

While somewhat perplexing by contemporary standards, several possibilities may account for why the WHO's leadership adopted this rather bizarre stance towards the notion of the SEP. One of the reasons proffered for why the bureaucracy was more committed to the MEP than the SEP has been that '[m]any of the leading figures in international public health during the 1960s had spent their formative years in vector control programmes, and it was with these that they were the most conversant and felt the most comfortable' (Fenner et al. 1988, p. 418). The implication of this observation is that because vector control programmes like the MEP focus on preventing disease transmission from animal hosts by eliminating the carrier of disease (namely the animal), the senior leadership of the WHO were uneasy about launching a global eradication campaign that targeted a disease such as smallpox which was only transmitted between humans. Likewise, while a freeze-dried version of the smallpox vaccine had recently been developed in Europe, its potential to replace the conventional vaccine (which, notably, was in short supply and required refrigeration to preserve it) was uncertain, as the new vaccine was still undergoing trials. Yet another possibility may simply have been that the WHO's resources were believed to be already stretched to their limit with the MEP, and the WHO's director-general was therefore reluctant to over-commit the fledgling IO. Finally, tensions between the USSR and the United States had also reached new heights in the early 1960s. It is therefore possible that the IO's senior leadership, conscious of these tensions, were reluctant to be perceived as enthusiastic about a project that was being heavily endorsed and supported by the USSR. Whichever the cause, the reality nevertheless became that even as international support emerged for the creation of an SEP special account to support the programme's implementation, the director-general sought to circumvent it becoming a reality (WHO 1966a, 1966b). Instead, it was maintained that the organization's primary focus should remain on conducting disease surveillance and the provision of quality-tested vaccines.

The IO's bureaucracy ultimately retained this non-interventionist stance towards smallpox eradication until the mid-1960s, when a series of internal and external factors forced it to become more involved. In January 1964, for example, Dr Karel Raska, a passionate advocate of smallpox eradication, was appointed Director of the Communicable Diseases Division. As head of this department, Dr Raska was able to successfully lobby the director-general to establish a Smallpox Eradication Unit within the WHO to provide support to those countries already undertaking eradication campaigns. Coinciding with Dr Raska's appointment, several of the more influential (proximal) principals, frustrated with the lack of progress, successfully managed to convince their compatriots to pass a new resolution in May 1964, calling on the WHO to develop a specific plan for achieving eradication as soon as possible – pressure they sustained through into the following year, scrutinizing the secretariat's progress to date and then calling for even further effort to be taken. Added to this, in 1965 the US president, Lyndon B. Johnson, publicly declared his country's firm support of the SEP and committed considerable resources to eradicating smallpox throughout western and central Africa – an area that, at the time, had increasingly become a focus of Cold War activities (WHO 1968a, Glynn and Glynn 2004). As a direct result of this additional political pressure, in 1965 the director-general presented a new nine-point strategy to the WHA detailing how smallpox eradication could be achieved (WHO 1965b). Yet while new impetus was beginning to emerge, much to the sustained frustration of its member states, the organization's senior bureaucracy continued to procrastinate, undertaking further reviews that sought to assess the long-term viability of the programme.

Despite the WHO's senior leadership's apparent reluctance at this time, a confluence of events nevertheless occurred in the mid-1960s that, as will be discussed below, soon resulted in a transformation in the IO's management of the SEP. It can be observed, for example, that the creation of the Smallpox Eradication Unit and the appointment of Dr Karel Raska as its head created a bureaucratic cluster of like-minded individuals committed to the goal of smallpox eradication within the WHO – in effect, an epistemic community that achieved a particular prominence and influence within the IO. At the exact same time, external to the WHO, Dr Donald Henderson was appointed as head of the surveillance section of the US Centre for Disease Control and Prevention (CDC). Henderson had spent a number of his formative years in medicine, working in smallpox eradication campaigns. Following the United States' declaration of support for the SEP, Henderson became instrumental in developing not only the US eradication strategy in West Africa, but he also contributed heavily to the re-evaluation of the WHO's global programme and strategy (WHO 1966c, Glynn and Glynn 2004). Later, by 1968, Henderson had been appointed the SEP's director, ensuring a direct link between the epistemic community within the WHO and one of the most influential (proximal) member states, the United States. These factors – the creation of an epistemic community within the WHO, the commitment of the United States, and the appointment of Dr Henderson and his involvement with, influence over, and subsequent leadership of the programme – arguably contributed to re-casting the senior WHO leadership's views towards smallpox eradication.

Indeed, by 1966 sufficient momentum had built to ensure the WHO would escalate its commitment to the eradication of smallpox, even if it was to do so without much enthusiasm. Although several senior WHO staff, including the director-general, continued to have profound reservations about the feasibility of eradicating the disease (Fenner et al. 1988), bowing to pressure from WHO member states (and possibly to pressure exerted from within the IO from the Smallpox Eradication Unit) the director-general arranged for a detailed report to be produced outlining how the programme could be advanced. In May 1966 this report was presented to the 19th WHA where it was then approved, and preparations were immediately undertaken for the launch of a second, intensified phase of the programme the following year.

The Intensified Smallpox Eradication Programme (ISEP) commenced on 1 January 1967 with the aim of achieving its objective of complete eradication within a decade. The strategy of the programme was essentially two-fold: firstly, to commence mass-vaccination programmes in all countries where smallpox was endemic using high-quality freeze-dried vaccines; and secondly, to develop and maintain an effective surveillance and detection system to identify individual cases and contain larger outbreaks. In light of the increasingly evident failure of the MEP, and to the WHO bureaucracy's credit, three principles were also recognized to be particularly important in guiding the ISEP's implementation. The first of these was that if complete eradication was to be achieved, all countries needed to participate in the programme. Secondly, the WHO decided that considerable flexibility would be afforded to individual national campaigns in order that they may adapt to local social, cultural, and practical conditions. Thirdly, based on its experiences of resistance to DDT, the WHO agreed that ongoing research would be required to discover new innovative methods for achieving eradication.

In fact, there is clear evidence to support the observation that by the time the intensified phase of the SEP commenced the WHO's bureaucracy had 'learned' a number of important lessons from the failures of the MEP and several other disease eradication campaigns. In one internal document outlining the new SEP strategy that was to be followed, for instance, it was openly acknowledged that '[t]he particular lesson learned has been that it is preferable for the general health services to be involved from the start rather than to wait for years (as in the case of earlier yaws control and BCG vaccination programmes) before integration is attempted' (WHO 1966d, p. 1, emphasis original). Likewise, in an acknowledgement of the WHO's past inflexibility in eradication programmes, Dr Raska himself noted in a 1966 speech presented to the IX International Congress for Microbiology:

> It is also impossible to use for the whole world one too simplified recommendation about vaccination coverage. Logistics in planning, implementation, surveillance and continuous assessment of the programme and necessary flexibility to react in a proper epidemiological way in any unexpected situation should correspond to the different ecological and socio-economic conditions in a given country or groups of countries. (WHO 1966e, p. 5)

In addition to this acknowledgement, the WHO took a much more proactive approach to the technical assistance it offered. Key to this capability was the Smallpox Eradication Unit, which, as Henderson (1987b, p. 543) notes, 'took an active operational role rather than serving in the more common advisory technical capacity. Being in frequent contact with national and WHO programme staff, the unit could anticipate problems, evaluate requests and respond quickly'. The benefits of this new strategy were manifest, as Henderson observes:

> The smallpox eradication unit in WHO headquarters established a central point of contact for those outside the programme, whether scientists, potential donors, candidates to join the staff, or the media. Because the unit kept abreast of and widely disseminated the current technical information on smallpox, there was regular communication between the professional staff and the scientific and public health communities. This facilitated the rapid translation into practice of new developments. (ibid., p. 541)

It is therefore not surprising that Fenner and colleagues (1988, p. 380) have correspondingly argued, with reference to the MEP, that the 'successes and failures of its policies provided guidance in formulating [the] smallpox eradication strategy'; and go on to make the case that the intensified phase of the SEP differed from the MEP in three notable ways. Firstly, the WHO only sought to provide generic principles for how countries could pursue smallpox eradication, avoiding the highly prescriptive format it had adopted throughout the MEP. This allowed countries to amend their respective eradication campaigns to meet local conditions and requirements. In addition, the reporting and surveillance system was introduced much earlier into each campaign's operational phase, allowing member states to use epidemic intelligence to respond rapidly to new outbreaks before the attack phase of the their campaign was completed. Small outbreaks were therefore often able to be prevented from transforming into larger outbreaks or epidemics. Finally, in direct contrast to the MEP that assumed one strategy was sufficient to achieve eradication, the ISEP also promoted the idea that research and new methods of achieving eradication should be actively pursued. The IO's adoption of these three principles thus represented a significant leap in the WHO's governance methodology, and in the years to follow, they began to manifest in a number of very beneficial ways.

In 1967, for example, the WHO produced a manual to ensure SEP personnel possessed sufficient awareness of the programme's overall policies and procedures. Yet in stark contrast to the MEP, where health authorities were expected to implement the organization's policies wholesale and without deviation, SEP staff were actually encouraged to be innovative. It was explicitly acknowledged, for instance, in the handbook's foreword:

> that no manual could provide a satisfactory single blue-print which could be universally applicable, considering the many smallpox endemic countries and the vast differences in present health structures, personnel and policies, population characteristics and attitudes, geography and climate. (WHO 1967b, p. 1)

Moreover, although no future versions of the WHO manual were ever actually produced, the 1967 version was purposefully distributed in 'draft' form because the organization's bureaucracy had developed the view that '[a] Manual such as this must continually evolve as the global programme progresses and must constantly be subjected to query and criticism' (ibid.). This signalled a distinct change in the organization's attitude and overall approach to disease eradication projects, with the WHO's bureaucracy functioning more as a policy *adviser*, allowing national health authorities to deviate from the organization's recommendations without fear of financial reprisals accompanying their decision.

In fact, the only element that the WHO did maintain as essential to every national eradication campaign was the need to conduct comprehensive disease surveillance. Even in this though, the WHO bureaucracy approached the issue in a qualitatively different manner compared to its actions throughout the MEP. Firstly, whereas the organization had emphasized the importance of surveillance throughout the MEP, from 1967 onwards the WHO advocated that disease surveillance was 'the single most important component of the present global eradication effort' (WHO 1968b, p. 2). Evidencing the considerable weight the IO attached to this activity the WHO then arranged, upon request, for mobile surveillance teams to conduct on-site visits to local eradication units in each country. This in turn had a noticeable impact upon how the activity was perceived more generally. As Henderson (1977, p. 89) has observed, '[t]he fact that someone was actively interested in receiving reports and, moreover, took action on the basis of such reports was a new and unique experience for local health staff in many countries'. Correspondingly, a new ethos emerged, one that permeated the entire global effort as Henderson again later noted:

> the primary goal of the programme was 0 cases of smallpox and not X millions of vaccinations. Each case which occurred thus implied a weakness or failure in the programme. Knowledge of how and where such failures occurred permitted continuing modification in the programme so as to permit the optimal deployment of resources where they could be most effective. (ibid., p. 87)

The WHO's revised disease eradication tactics extended beyond disease surveillance into the broader operational context though as well. For instance, in the opening months of 1973 a number of epidemics broke out in India, Bangladesh, and Pakistan, the scale of which had not been observed since the commencement of the programme in 1959. National authorities aided by WHO specialists responded rapidly, instigating a variety of containment measures to suppress the epidemics. Nevertheless, it was determined that to prevent further outbreaks from emerging, closer and more prompt detection of index cases was required. The national authorities thus amended their respective campaign strategies to include door-to-door searches engaging volunteers, community groups, and health workers alike, and offering substantial monetary rewards (derived from WHO-administered funds) when cases were reported.[4] This combination of measures proved to be very effective in detecting new cases of smallpox before they developed into major outbreaks, and transmission was ultimately halted in these countries between 1974 and 1975.

Of course, on the converse side, not every decision taken by the WHO proved beneficial. One example that was shown to be particularly obstructive was the determination by the director-general to prevent any re-allocation of regional SEP funds. This verdict prevented funds being moved from regional areas that had already eradicated smallpox to other regions that had yet to do so. Consequently, while the director-general's decision was made on the basis of political expediency,[5] the implication was that funds that could have been made available to assist countries achieve eradication were not. Another related instance emerged from the strict accounting requirements in the dispensing and allocation of funds at the national level. Although this was later able to be resolved by the WHO taking an innovative approach and establishing 'impress accounts' for staff, strict accounting practices at the commencement of the programme were observed to negatively impact upon a variety of operational issues such as travel arrangements of field staff and petrol and maintenance allowances for SEP-dedicated vehicles (Henderson 1987b, pp. 543–544).

Nevertheless, despite several of these decision-making mishaps, it can be discerned that the governance approach adopted by the WHO bureaucracy throughout the ISEP was substantially different from the methodology it had employed in the context of the MEP. Moreover, this different style of governance influenced the roles that the WHO was prepared and able to effect. For example, throughout the ISEP the WHO functioned more as a policy adviser rather than prescriber: member states were free to choose whether or not they would adhere by the WHO's policies, and were able to make their decision without any fear that the financial support for their respective national campaigns would be withdrawn as a result of that decision. While the IO continued to exercise its normative power to coerce national health authorities into following the WHO's policies wherever it could, the organization was unable and – more significantly – unwilling to compel member states to do so.

The WHO bureaucracy was observed to approach its epidemic intelligence activities very differently as well. For instance, in contrast to the MEP, the WHO encouraged member states to undertake disease surveillance much earlier and report more regularly. This data was then used by the organization to assist member states and, wherever possible, to respond to local outbreaks while simultaneously informing the development of the global SEP policy. The intelligence the WHO received also enabled the bureaucracy to promote the need for new innovative research, as trials were reported and evaluated more efficiently. The WHO thus functioned more as a coordinator of the epidemic intelligence it received, using the information to guide and promote new developments and progress with the overall success of the programme, rather than merely consolidating the information as it had done throughout the MEP. Moreover, although occasionally the IO's detached oversight was observed to result in minor difficulties emerging between WHO personnel and national health authorities (particularly when local or government health officials were involved in attempting to conceal smallpox outbreaks),[6] generally the atmosphere was one of collegiality, cooperation, and equality – an environment that was qualitatively unlike the MEP.

Equally, the WHO's management of the SEP was defined by an absence of at least one role that it had performed throughout the MEP: that of government assessor. In large part, this was accomplished by the fact that funding and technical assistance was not linked to a requirement for countries to adhere to WHO policies. Rather, from the very start of the global campaign the organization actively sought to distance itself by insisting that each member state was answerable for the expenses, administration, and execution of its respective operations. Later, once the SEP special account had been established and the intensified phase of the programme began, technical assistance and funding was made available to states upon request and without censure – even, notably, as evidence began to emerge of member states falsifying vaccination records, thereby jeopardizing the success of the entire campaign (Glynn and Glynn 2004, pp. 202–206). The bureaucracy instead sought to promote a collaborative approach to eradication, encouraging the view that even one case of smallpox was a failure of all parties, not just the government of the territory concerned.

Indeed, even from the launch of the first stage of the programme, the WHO approached the entire global campaign to eradicate smallpox very differently – an approach that undoubtedly contributed to the international community achieving its final objective of the Smallpox Target Zero campaign (Henderson 1977, p. 87).[7] Of course, it is now widely accepted that the smallpox virus was a more conducive candidate for eradication than malaria, particularly given that, as Henderson (ibid., p. 86) has noted, 'the clinical and epidemiological characteristics of smallpox were unusually favourable for eradication; a remarkably effective vaccine was available; and, universally, there was greater concern about smallpox than any other communicable disease'. At the same time, however, as evidenced by the discussion above, the flexible governance approach adopted by the WHO throughout the SEP also arguably contributed to the success of the campaign – a campaign that remains to this day widely regarded as one of the WHO's greatest achievements. Testifying to this, it is important to note that at the beginning of the programme some 60 per cent of the world's population lived in smallpox-endemic countries. Yet by the end of a 10-year, 10-month intensified campaign the IO witnessed the complete eradication of a disease that had persisted in afflicting humanity for over three millennia. Donald Henderson, the intensified programme's director, later commented that much of the SEP's achievements could be attributed to the organization's accommodating management approach (Henderson 1987b), while the former director-general, Dr Haflan Mahler, was quoted as having stated that the SEP was 'a triumph of management, not of medicine' (quoted in Hopkins 1989, p. 125). Although management alone cannot account for the success of the SEP, the WHO did learn several very valuable lessons – lessons that it has continued to apply to future global disease eradication programmes and control efforts, including its Global TB Programme.

The WHO and TB

Alongside malaria, TB was identified by the founders of the WHO as being one amongst a cluster of diseases that required urgent attention by the newly created health agency. Until relatively recently though, the WHO's overall efforts in addressing the TB threat could be characterized by something akin to remote disinterest. As will be discussed below, several factors can arguably account for the development of this state of affairs. While it is important to appreciate that the IO cannot be held entirely to blame for its past neglect of this disease, it is necessary to examine past trends and developments to appreciate the WHO's current involvement and how it came about. This section therefore seeks to provide a brief historical overview of both the WHO's involvement in responding to TB and the constraints that the organization has faced throughout this period.

At the close of WWII, TB epidemics had become a common feature throughout many of the post-conflict regions of the world. It should not be surprising, therefore, that the management of this disease was viewed by the WHO Interim Commission as a matter of considerable importance. Certainly, while discussions pertaining to the control of malaria dominated much of the Interim Commission's initial deliberations, determining the organization's role in responding to the ongoing, widespread, and 'rampant' TB epidemics was identified as an issue that required immediate consideration as early as the Commission's second meeting (WHO 1947c, p. 21). Dr Andre Cavaillon, the director-general of the French Ministry of Health, later summed up the view of most delegates, stating '[t]he problem of tuberculosis was of worldwide importance, and the future WHO would be judged by its attitude to it' (WHO 1948d, p. 13). Evidently the members of the Interim Commission concurred, as they soon established the WHO Expert Committee on Tuberculosis and instigated the organization's first official engagement with managing TB in January 1948.

It was in this regard that the IO's first practical response to the resurgence of post-war TB was to initiate a joint project with UNICEF, focusing particularly on preventing the disease's further dissemination throughout Europe. The central strategy of the campaign built on the concurrent work being undertaken by the Danish Red Cross in Poland, which focused on vaccinating children with the Bacille Calmette-Guérin (BCG) vaccine. Supplementing this strategy, the WHO also initiated a series of surveys or disease surveillance activities to assist countries in allocating sufficient personnel and resources to deal with new TB cases. Yet while the campaign lasted some three and a half years and vaccinated some 18 million children throughout 23 countries, serious questions began to emerge regarding the BCG vaccine and whether it realistically afforded any protection against TB. Consequently, the WHO and the other agencies engaged in anti-TB efforts amended their prevention strategies and, with the emergence of new antibiotic therapies to treat the disease, began to target active cases of TB instead of merely vaccinating populations.

By the early 1950s the emergence and proven efficiency of antibiotic therapies literally revolutionized the way TB was seen as a disease. New trials of combination therapies (conducted mostly in developed countries) were soon demonstrating that TB sufferers could be successfully treated in outpatient clinics and even in their own homes. As a result, within the space of a decade the sanatoriums that had persisted as the dominant method of treating TB patients were being closed down in the majority of industrialized countries. WHO-supported national anti-TB campaigns began to flourish. Yet even as TB infections became increasingly rare throughout Europe and North America, in the developing world infections continued unabated, largely due to the fact that the costs associated with combination chemotherapy treatment were prohibitive. As the WHO director-general recorded in 1952 in a rather remarkable admission:

> Experience of the tuberculosis projects during the year confirmed the belief that many of the control methods and techniques used in the more developed countries cannot be successfully transplanted to other parts of the world. WHO's objective in the control of

tuberculosis must be to assist each country to find the method most suited to its own particular conditions, to demonstrate these methods and to train its national personnel accordingly. (Quoted in Calder 1958, p. 23)

Thus, even though the WHO Expert Committee on Tuberculosis later declared in 1960 that the disease 'should receive priority and emphasis both by WHO and by governments' and that it was 'generally conceded to be the most important specific communicable disease in the world as a whole' (WHO 1960d, p. 4), international efforts to control TB effectively stalled as a number of the more wealthy donors – namely the industrialized countries – lost interest.

By the late 1970s TB was no longer viewed as a significant public health issue by the majority of Western countries. While drug-resistant cases of TB had been infrequently observed to emerge, the array of effective treatment options had also been intermittently expanded with the creation of new antibiotics. Throughout the industrialized world, eradicating TB therefore simply began to be perceived as a matter of ensuring adequate supplies of drugs – something that the majority of Western countries had no difficulty in securing. Correspondingly, with the added realization of the failure of the MEP and the 1970s economic crisis prompting substantial re-structuring of healthcare more generally (Chorev 2012), financial contributions for WHO-supported national anti-TB campaigns began to dissipate and interest in TB as a public health issue waned.

The emergence of the HIV in the 1980s and multi-drug-resistant tuberculosis (MDRTB) in the 1990s ultimately revealed, however, just how disastrous the policy of neglecting TB programmes and developing new treatments would become. Indeed new strains of TB, comingling with HIV and/or arising from individuals' non-compliance with anti-TB medications, soon presented a variety of new challenges for the medical establishment as conventional treatments were shown to be ineffective. As a result, by the early 1990s TB had once again begun to spread extensively throughout many Western developed countries. Meanwhile, the WHO's policies had remained unchanged for more than two decades and, disturbingly, the organization's capacity to respond to the resurgence was at an all-time low due to the reality that the control programmes previously initiated in the 1960s and 1970s had been gradually and systematically scaled back through lack of financial support (Raviglione and Pio 2002). In fact, by the time TB was re-appearing as a concern amongst Western interests again, the IO's contingent of

TB-dedicated personnel had diminished to just two staff members (Cegielski et al. 2002). Suddenly unacceptable to several of the more influential member states (and especially the developed countries whose populations were now under renewed threat), the issue of controlling TB was once again granted renewed status within the organization and a new initiative was launched to address the recently re-discovered global threat.

In 1991, in recognition of the danger that TB presented to the entire international community, the 44th WHA announced its intention to increase anti-TB efforts and proclaimed that every national TB programme should pursue two central objectives (see resolution WHA44.8 in WHO 1993a). Firstly, the WHA decreed that every country should aim to detect at least 70 per cent of all smear-positive or active TB cases. Secondly, it declared that every national programme should allocate sufficient resources to successfully treat 85 per cent of all cases detected. Highlighting the renewed importance the international community attached to the control of TB, every member state was also encouraged to achieve these objectives by the year 2000, and the WHO was correspondingly expected to assist countries in this endeavour. As noted above, however, the organization's capacity was noticeably constrained in this regard. The extent of the WHO's assistance at this time was therefore limited to supporting national campaigns through the provision of training materials and guidelines while also seeking to coordinate new international research in such areas as discovering new case detection techniques and treatment options.

By 1993, in response to the renewed interest by developed countries and especially the United States, the WHO's director-general prepared a report on the global situation and presented it to the 46th WHA. The statistics detailed in the report were alarming: one third of the world's population was believed to be infected with TB; eight million new cases were thought to emerge every year; some three million deaths per year were estimated to be attributable to TB; and 95 per cent of all of these cases occurred in the developing world. Noting that TB was 'thus a major global health problem', the director-general stated:

> This tragic situation continues even though a strategy exists to control tuberculosis and the tools for its implementation, though not yet perfect, are available. Past neglect by governments in all regions, misunderstanding of the methods and potential for disease control and a veering of scientific and research interests away from infectious diseases that are no longer important in the industrialized world

and from the health problems of poor developing societies where tuberculosis remains rife, explain but cannot excuse this situation. (WHO 1993b, p. 148)

To add weight to the report and in an attempt to engender a greater allocation of resources to tackle the disease, the WHO had announced just one month earlier the resurgence of TB to be a 'global emergency' (WHO 1994). Unfortunately though, even with a state of emergency having been declared, the WHO's attempts to embarrass the international community (and particularly the more wealthy developed states) into committing more resources failed, and progress in tackling the disease remained slow.

For example, one of the key strategies endorsed by the 44th WHA that then began to be widely promoted by the WHO's bureaucracy was the Directly Observed Treatment, Short-course (DOTS). Originally derived from anti-TB work undertaken in India in the 1950s, the DOTS strategy has since emerged to become *the* central strategy of the international community's TB control campaign. At its most basic, DOTS aims to fortify political and financial support; promote case-detection through quality-assured bacteriology; ensure standardized treatment that is supervised and supportive of patients; establish an effective drug supply and management system; and ensure continual monitoring, evaluation, and impact assessments (WHO 2002a, pp. 116–119). Yet while the strategy was endorsed by the WHA in 1991, by 1995 only 35 per cent of the world's governments had actually begun to implement DOTS, and only 18 per cent were able to claim they had made the programme available countrywide (Raviglione et al. 1997, p. 627). Similarly, it was only in 1995 that the WHO was able to obtain sufficient funds to establish a new international surveillance and monitoring project to evaluate the progress made by national TB control programmes in implementing DOTS.

It is equally important to note, however, that the WHO's difficulties in securing additional resources from member states at this time was not without some cause. Indeed, by the mid-1990s a number of influential member states had lost confidence in the organization's ability to manage infectious diseases effectively. This crisis of confidence had arisen in part from the IO's negligence of HIV/AIDS, which had in turn prompted the international community to establish UNAIDS in 1996. In addition, a number of governments had lost faith in the WHO's director-general at the time, Dr Hiroshi Nakajima, who had become embroiled in accusations of corruption and nepotism. Subsequently, throughout the 1990s a variety of intergovernmental and non-governmental organizations, institutions, and agencies had begun to directly challenge the WHO's normative leadership role and its technical efforts in international health work; and the crisis of confidence exacerbated the organization's existing economic and technical constraints.

In an attempt to focus global attention on the TB 'emergency', the WHO in collaboration with several other partner organizations launched the Stop TB Initiative in March 1998. By working together with a wide variety of interested parties that included governments, non-governmental organizations (NGOs), and private sector organizations, the Initiative sought to generate greater awareness about the TB emergency and thereby trigger greater political commitment and resources. In effect, the Initiative's purpose was thus to ensure not only the more effective coordination of existing resources, but also the mobilization of more resources to address the TB emergency in developed and developing countries. The culmination of the Initiative's work in this area was the Ministerial Conference on Tuberculosis and Sustainable Development held in March 2000 in Amsterdam, The Netherlands, where participating member states gave several new assurances and set a number of new goals to confront the disease. Hailed as 'a defining moment in the restructuring of global efforts to control TB' (Riccardi et al. 2009, p. 608), the Amsterdam conference also proposed the creation of a new global partnership to eliminate TB and the further expansion of the DOTS strategy. Momentum correspondingly began to build; and the Ministerial Conference was then followed by a series of prominent intergovernmental ministerial meetings held between 2000 and 2001. Recognizing that the original objective of the year 2000 was unattainable, the international community subsequently developed several new targets that aimed to reduce the global burden of TB by the year 2015. The primary international vehicle that was purpose-built to advance the international community's efforts in this endeavour is the Stop TB Partnership.

The Stop TB Partnership was created in October 2001 with the primary objective of eliminating TB as a public health threat. Currently comprising approximately 1,000 agencies, institutions, foundations, governments, organizations, and individuals, the Partnership aims to bring together interested parties based on their capacity and willingness to contribute to the goal of halving TB prevalence and fatality rates worldwide by 2015, using 1990 figures as a baseline (Stop TB Partnership 2006). To achieve this, the Partnership established a number of working groups to provide direction and guidance in areas such as expanding the DOTS strategy; developing new diagnostic tools to detect TB cases; advancing research to develop new TB drugs and vaccines; ensuring that there are sufficient mechanisms in place to tackle MDRTB and TB/HIV coinfection issues; and general advocacy, communications, and social mobilization. It is important to note, however, that while the Partnership is categorized as an independent entity, the WHO forms an integral component of this regime.

For instance, the Partnership's administrative element, the Stop TB Secretariat, is housed within the WHO headquarters in Geneva and forms part of the organization's Stop TB Department. This decision taken by the Partnership was specifically intended 'to facilitate collaboration with the WHO, to benefit from the WHO's robust infrastructure and international legitimacy' (Kumaresan et al. 2004, p. 126). In addition, the secretariat is subject to 'the rules and regulations of WHO for its administrative, financial and human resources management' except, that is, where alterations are deemed necessary to meet the specific needs of the Stop TB Partnership (Stop TB Partnership 2004, p. 14).

Further, the WHO remains responsible for coordinating the development of all global strategy and policy in relation to TB control – strategies and policies that the Stop TB Partnership then executes. Chief among these has been the WHO's work in relation to DOTS. For the past decade and a half the IO has been at the forefront of promoting the implementation of the DOTS strategy throughout high-burden, TB-endemic countries. In more recent years the DOTS strategy has had to undergo revision in order to ensure that it is responsive to the growing challenges of MDRTB and TB/HIV, and the WHO has been responsible for developing new initiatives such as the DOTS Plus programme to tackle these issues. Alongside this activity, the organization is responsible for coordinating the Partnership's working group on expanding the DOTS strategy and overseeing the Global DOTS Expansion Plan (GDEP) through which the WHO has been actively engaged in promoting the creation of coalitions between national health authorities, and local, regional, and international partners to address the needs of individual countries. Understandably, the WHO has therefore played *the* leading role in setting the international community's TB-control targets; but it has functioned as a coordinating agency, issuing recommendations and guidance documents that member states are encouraged (but not obliged) to implement.

It is also arguable that in this regard the Stop TB Partnership has adopted the same ethos that the WHO displayed following the failure of the MEP. The Partnership has explicitly stated, for instance:

Effective TB control cannot be imposed from above. It is a fundamental premise of the *Global Plan to Stop TB* that national governments and local communities take responsibility for planning and implementing their TB-prevention and treatment programmes. (Stop TB Partnership 2001, p. 15, emphasis original)

Although the Stop TB Secretariat thus coordinates and supports the Partnership's approximately 1,000 members engaged in TB control programmes – in effect creating an epistemic community of like-minded individuals committed to a common cause – individual governments remain accountable for their own campaign's execution and ongoing maintenance. The Partnership's policy thereby mirrors and reinforces the WHO's now standard position that the IO will coordinate international efforts while simultaneously seeking to deflect responsibility for them.

Likewise, the WHO has remained the central actor involved in collating and disseminating TB-related epidemic intelligence. Although this is a function that the organization has performed since its foundation, particularly since the mid-1990s the organization has been heavily involved in the collection and analysis of worldwide TB trends, producing a variety of reports and information documents for international dissemination. In more recent years, this has been augmented by the WHO's development of an interactive global TB database that permits interested parties the opportunity to examine the latest data on prevalence rates and expected fatalities, including country-specific profiles and high-risk areas. The WHO has been able to retain this central role through its close links with member states and the comprehensive network of WHO-affiliated surveillance laboratories and treatment centres. The Stop TB Partnership is thereby reliant upon the data obtained and processed by the organization to inform its own policy choices. Correspondingly, the WHO exists as *the* international community's recognized authority in TB-related epidemic intelligence.

It can be observed, therefore, that the WHO's relationship with the Stop TB Partnership is interdependent, complex, and multidimensional. At the same time, however, both entities remain ostensibly independent. For while the IO is expected to provide the Partnership with general guidance and may recommend that it adopt certain policies and procedures, it is the Partnership's Coordinating Board – which lists the WHO as merely one member amongst 34 other partners, including governments, private institutions, organizations, foundations, and individuals – that makes the final determination. Similarly, while the Stop TB Secretariat continues to be housed within the WHO and is answerable to the IO's director-general, the secretariat is responsible for coordinating general administration, finance, communication, and advocacy. The secretariat also independently manages the Global TB Drug Facility (GDF) that provides TB drugs on a short-term basis to countries. The GDF thereby facilitates the further expansion of the DOTS strategy – one of the tasks that falls under the jurisdiction of the WHO. It is in this regard that the Global Partnership's governance model is considered to be 'successfully balanced' as it 'has been carefully calibrated to ensure representation of the diverse constituencies' while recognizing 'the need for consensus with the need for decisive rapid action' (Kumaresan et al. 2004, p. 126).

This arrangement between the Stop TB Partnership and the WHO is therefore particularly unusual when compared to the IO's past efforts at eradicating infectious disease threats. For instance, through its involvement with the Partnership the WHO is only currently engaged in an attempt to eliminate TB as a public health threat. While this objective incorporates the ideal of eradication, it simultaneously retreats from firmly committing to the principle. This is particularly significant when considering a second factor, namely that the WHO has essentially delegated its disease eradication responsibilities to a third, independent party. For while the organization has, and will likely continue to maintain, a prominent role in the overall global campaign, equally, the WHO is technically no longer directly responsible for ensuring that TB is eradicated. Notably, however, this is in marked contrast to the IO's obligations as required by its constitution. Given these factors and the remarkable dissimilarities between the WHO's efforts in relation to TB and its former disease eradication campaigns such as the MEP and SEP, it is reasonable to ask: Can the WHO be considered to have developed a classical approach to disease eradication?

The classical approach examined

Even from the brief overview provided above, it is reasonable to conclude that the organization's bureaucracy has developed a classical approach to managing infectious diseases. This is principally because while some differences may be discernible in relation to the technical responses of each campaign – for instance, the level and extent of technical assistance provided, the nature of the policy advice supplied, and the technical measures adopted depending on how the disease is transmitted (i.e. vector-borne, air-borne, or transmitted by bodily fluids) – a clear pattern has nevertheless emerged in the aftermath of the MEP in terms of the governance methodology employed by the WHO.

This methodology is categorized by a number of features. Most notably, following the unqualified failure of the MEP the WHO has consistently eschewed and shirked opportunities to act as the international community's directing authority in international health matters. Instead, as the cases above have illustrated, since the MEP the organization's bureaucracy has unswervingly sought to function more as a coordinating agency or facilitator, encouraging member states to take ownership and responsibility for their own respective disease eradication campaigns. While in some ways this new approach was consistent with the authority envisaged by the WHO's founders, two factors in particular arguably contributed to the bureaucracy amending the IO's governance style: the collapse of the MEP and member states' subsequent decision to rein in the organization through their control mechanisms.

It was immediately apparent in 1958, for example, that the WHO's bureaucracy was disinclined to launch yet another global eradication campaign – the SEP. Although several political, technical, and logistical considerations may have assisted in explaining this initial reluctance, by the mid- to late 1960s the bureaucracy's concern appears to have shifted to the possibility that the smallpox programme would prove to be yet another momentous failure like the MEP that would, in turn, damage its reputation as an effective and efficient IO. The programme's economic constraints, which persisted well into the final stages of the campaign and were driven by donors' recent experiences with the failed MEP, also arguably reinforced the WHO's seemingly nonchalant attitude towards the initiative. As a result, however, even as the organization embarked on the intensified phase of the global smallpox campaign, the bureaucracy maintained that while it would assist member states, governments were to be ultimately responsible for their own national eradication campaigns and the policies they chose to implement (such as mandatory vaccinations). Wherever necessary and upon request, the IO would provide technical assistance and financial support to ensure national campaigns were aware of the latest eradication techniques and programme developments. But it was made equally clear to each country that it was responsible for the administration and execution of the campaign in its territory. In part by choice and in part by compulsion, therefore, in fulfilling its health-for-security delegation contract the WHO's bureaucracy embraced its role as a coordinating agency, working to synchronize the international community's efforts to successfully achieve the eradication of smallpox.

In contrast, in the context of the WHO's TB campaign, a firm commitment was originally demonstrated for the IO's bureaucracy to work towards the eradication of the disease. Yet through a combination of events – including the development of new technologies such as antibiotics, disillusionment with the WHO's past performance, and a global economic crisis – a number of influential member states lost interest in pursuing this goal. The WHO's TB activities were thus left in limbo, and even deliberately downgraded, until such time as Western developed countries were (re)awoken to the threat TB presented. Further, even though the organization's bureaucracy then displayed its willingness to go to extraordinary lengths, conspicuously declaring a global emergency to tackle this disease, member states chose to bypass the IO and create a new international regime to lead the charge: the Stop TB Partnership, which in turn was ultimately overshadowed by the Global Fund to Fight AIDS, TB and Malaria. The WHO thus again functioned largely as a facilitator, operating behind the scenes in developing global policy and providing the means for the Stop TB Partnership to achieve its objective of eliminating TB as a public health threat.

Further, as the above illustrations have testified, even as the WHO bureaucracy progressively sought to give effect to its health-for-security mandate, there were limits to which the IO was prepared (and permitted) to perform. For instance, it is apparent that one of the key functions the WHO has reliably performed since its creation has been the collection and collation of epidemic intelligence. In its first days of operation, though, the organization's bureaucracy largely regurgitated the information it obtained, melding the data into guidelines and procedures that were then to be implemented without deviation – functioning, in effect, as an epidemic intelligence consolidator. However, after the disintegration of the MEP, the organization recognized the unsuitability of such practices and began to use the information it received to evaluate and critically reflect on the policies it was promoting. This marked a distinct change in the IO's modus operandi, with the bureaucracy seeking to behave more as an epidemic intelligence coordinator of the data it received, identifying gaps in existing knowledge, promoting new research, and providing, wherever possible, recommendations based on sound evidence.

Following closely behind the organization's transformation in relation to epidemic intelligence, the WHO also began to act more as a policy adviser in the wake of the MEP, as opposed to acting as the international community's policy prescriber. It may be recalled, for example, that the WHO bureaucracy had initially adopted a very prescriptive, authoritarian attitude in relation to the MEP policies it formulated. The collapse of the malaria programme again revealed how ill-advised this outlook had been; and correspondingly, the bureaucracy began to encourage not only its staff, but also member states and national health authorities to adapt its policies where they were identified to be ineffective. The bureaucracy, in essence, became more flexible in its approach, and while the policies the WHO produced were increasingly based on the latest available evidence, the IO continued to stress their status as recommendations rather than directives. This proved a very timely change for the intensified phase of the SEP, as it permitted member states to adapt their campaign structure and operational activities to address local conditions. Likewise, this change has encouraged member states to revise their TB control strategies where evidence indicates that the former methods are not working.

The third – and arguably the most significant – change was that the WHO bureaucracy has, since the MEP, systematically and unfailingly avoided functioning as a government assessor. Throughout the malaria campaign the WHO bureaucracy was observed to scrutinize member states' compliance with its policies, and where deviations were noted WHO personnel were made available to assist member states remedy them. Further, although the bureaucracy itself was not responsible for donors choosing to withhold funds from those countries not adhering to the organization's policies, by failing to condemn the action the bureaucracy tacitly signalled its endorsement of the practice. Similarly, during the MEP's operation select member states had been excluded from the programme on the basis of technical and political considerations with the full knowledge and consent of the WHO's leadership.

In the context of both the global campaign to eradicate smallpox and the Stop TB programme though, the WHO bureaucracy has sought, as much as possible, to avoid repeating these practices. To begin with, the organization has gone to (and continues to go to) considerable lengths to ensure that no country is excluded from its global campaigns, whether the aim is simply control (i.e. TB) or the more substantial goal of eradication (smallpox, polio, and similar diseases). In fact, where countries have been noted to distance themselves from engaging in such campaigns, the WHO's bureaucracy has sought to use every available means at its disposal to encourage their participation. At the same time, the organization has returned to the system envisaged by the WHO's founders of only assisting member states upon request, signifying its respect for member states' sovereignty and the principle of non-interference. Thus even though member states regularly diverged from the WHO's procedures throughout the SEP, in contrast to the malaria campaign this divergence was actively encouraged by the IO's bureaucracy – a feature that was also promoted in eliminating TB.

Yet another feature of the WHO's classical approach to managing infectious diseases is that the IO's bureaucracy has painstakingly sought to avoid even the perception that it criticizes its member states. In part, this practice has developed from a recognition of the innate importance of the organization's own reputation as an efficient and effective IO. The WHO bureaucracy has, perhaps understandably, therefore become extremely protective of its status and has habitually sought to avoid any situation that may reflect poorly on its performance and/or attract criticism. Equally, however, the bureaucracy has stringently avoided being perceived as criticizing its member states due to the potential (unwelcome) repercussions that may result from such an incident – for example, the imposition of further politico-legal, economic, technical, or socio-legal constraints. Said another way, member states have successfully managed to make it clear to the WHO bureaucracy that there are significant limitations on the IO's role, authority, and autonomy. In order to achieve its primary mission and continue to remain relevant to the wider international community, the organization must cooperate with member states. Subsequently the WHO bureaucracy is reluctant to engage in any activity, or be perceived to be engaging in any activity, that may jeopardize its relationship with its principals.

Finally, throughout each of the WHO's global disease eradication campaigns the IO has rarely functioned as the international community's lead technical agency. Instead the organization has preferred to allow its member states to initiate any requests for the IO to intervene, often waiting for the WHA to pass resolutions that effectively compel the bureaucracy to act. It is likely this trend has arisen in part due to an acknowledgement by the bureaucracy of the IO's limited autonomy and an awareness of member states' mechanisms of control – most notably the economic constraints. At the same time, however, and as attested to by the IO's negligence of the HIV/AIDS threat, the WHO has also occasionally failed to assume the lead in combating infectious diseases even though member states have demanded that it do so. Whether or not these instances may be classified as examples of the WHO shirking its delegation contract, the result has been that the organization has seldom acted as the world's lead agency as originally envisaged.

Conclusion

Part I of this book has highlighted that the WHO was established with the specific purpose of ensuring the highest possible level of health for all peoples. Intrinsic to that purpose is the eradication of infectious diseases, and the organization was correspondingly invested with a considerable degree of authority and autonomy when it was first created to execute that duty. In effect, this formed an embedded disease eradication delegation contract between the IO and its member states that outlines the broad parameters of association and interaction, while simultaneously signalling the obligation and sense of importance the WHO is to attribute to this function. Indeed, member states considered the WHO's health-for-security role via eradicating infectious diseases to be so significant that they were willing to permit the suspension of the IO's usual control mechanisms to deal with epidemics and other disease-related emergencies. The organization's role in working towards the eradication of all infectious diseases may thus be considered the WHO's foremost function amongst all of its delegated duties.

At the same time, member states were concerned that the newly created IO might exceed the parameters of its authority and as such, inserted several mechanisms of control into the organization's institutional design. These mechanisms, which fall under the broad taxonomy of politico-legal, economic, technical, and socio-legal measures, have effectively served to constrain the WHO bureaucracy from expanding its sphere of operation and competence, except where member states have explicitly permitted otherwise. While the WHO was therefore clearly intended to act as the directing and coordinating authority in the field of international health, and exist as the highest authority in that field, it is apparent that member states never anticipated that the IO's role, authority, and autonomy would be unlimited.

The WHO's duty to prevent, control, and eradicate infectious diseases was put to the test very early on in the organization's history. Unfortunately, the IO's first attempt at eradicating an infectious disease – malaria – proved a notable failure. But the WHO secretariat arguably learnt from this experience, applying several lessons learned to the smallpox eradication campaign and the attempts to control and eliminate TB. Through these experiences the WHO subsequently developed what may be considered a classical approach to managing infectious diseases. This approach is characterized by the organization's reluctance to act as a directing authority as well as two specific operational roles: epidemic intelligence coordinator and policy adviser. In the wake of the MEP's failure, the WHO bureaucracy has also gone to painstaking lengths to avoid even the perception that it is critical of its member states, fearful of the possible ramifications that engaging in such actions may bring. Finally, in contrast to its actions during the MEP, the WHO has also sought to engage every country in disease eradication and/or disease control campaigns so that it may function as an efficient and effective coordinating agency.

3
Securitization and SARS: A New Framing?

In many ways, the 2003 SARS outbreak was a remarkable event in the history of human interaction with infectious diseases. By the time the disease had been contained in July 2003, it had infected 8,422 people and caused the deaths of approximately 916 individuals (Huang 2011, see also WHO 2006a). Compared to numerous other infectious diseases at the time, such as malaria, HIV/AIDS, TB, and cholera, the human morbidity and mortality caused by the 2003 outbreak was relatively minor. Yet in some of the most affected areas the outbreak triggered social and political upheaval, and the global economic impact of the outbreak was estimated to have been between US$11 billion and US$100 billion (Asian Development Bank 2003, US GAO 2004).

For the WHO, the 2003 SARS outbreak also proved to be a remarkable event and powerfully illustrated the benefits of a new way of working. Indeed, as this chapter and the next go on to argue, by the time the SARS coronavirus had begun to spread internationally the WHO secretariat had come to embrace a new approach to managing infectious diseases that was increasingly being described as 'global health security'. Though not yet finalized, the IO's formal health-for-security delegation contract was undergoing a transformation – one in which health-for-security was being actively and intentionally recast. Health was no longer just viewed as a vehicle to ensure international peace and security, but instead had come to be recognized as a legitimate security issue in and of itself. This new understanding of health-as-security took some years for the WHO to fully embrace, but the timing of the SARS outbreak proved instrumental in convincing not only the IO's member states of the need for this new management style, but also several internal stakeholders within the organization.

This chapter examines the WHO's handling of the 2003 SARS outbreak and how through its management of the 2003 SARS outbreak the IO established a new standard in global disease outbreak alert and control. In so doing, the organization's secretariat also created new customary practices that (temporarily) reinterpreted the WHO's delegation contract. Although a number of governments, even individuals, made significant contributions to containing the SARS threat, given the focus of this book, attention has only been given to the actions of the IO, noting how the secretariat's management of the SARS-inspired crisis differed from the organization's classical approach to disease eradication. Prior to examining the WHO's response to the 2003 SARS outbreak though, it is important to spend a few moments contextualizing the environment in which the IO found itself.

The WHO in 2003

As discussed in the previous chapter, throughout the 1990s the WHO experienced a prolonged crisis of confidence relating to its overall effectiveness and continued relevance to the international community. One of the direct consequences of this crisis was that it aggravated the constraints under which the IO traditionally operated; as noted in the case of the WHO's anti-TB efforts, member states' perceptions can, and do, have a direct bearing on the effectiveness of the organization. By March 2003, however, the WHO was arguably a very different IO. In fact, the WHO was instead enjoying renewed support from amongst its member states and the international media: its relevance was no longer being questioned, and the organization was perceived to be competent, credible, and effective (Yamey 2002a, Yamey and Abbasi 2003). A number of factors can account for this turn of events, but ultimately one of the most significant contributing factors in improving the IO's reputation and standing was the appointment of Dr Gro Harlem Brundtland to the position of director-general in 1998.

Dr Brundtland was elected in May 1998 on a platform to reform the WHO. A former medical practitioner and prime minister of Norway who had been elected for three terms of office, Brundtland possessed the reputation of being an accomplished politician. Her involvement in the 1992 Rio Earth Summit also confirmed Brundtland's credentials as an effective international negotiator and campaigner. Given member states' prolonged disillusionment with the WHO's performance, Dr Brundtland's appointment was thus very much welcomed by both governments and the international media from the beginning, as the newly appointed director-general moved rapidly to fulfil her promise of reforming the WHO (Mach 1998).

Within two years of her appointment Brundtland had restructured the organization's bureaucratic composition, re-shaped its policies and strategic direction, and streamlined its activities. The WHO's multiple departments and programmes were consolidated into nine 'clusters', each headed by an executive director. These directors, along with Brundtland herself, formed a new inner cabinet to oversee and coordinate the activities of the organization and its six regional offices (WHO 1998a). A new corporate strategy was also then outlined in 1999, giving the IO a new strategic focus and indicating how accountability to its member states would be improved. Staff rotation programmes were introduced, and several senior bureaucratic positions were eliminated to reduce costs and make the overall structure less hierarchical. Although largely restricted to the WHO's central headquarters in Geneva, the reforms were extensive, well overdue, and generally viewed as an indication that the IO was finally on the path to becoming a more effective institution (Yamey 2002b). Member states reacted to Brundtland's reforms by significantly boosting their extrabudgetary funds, and by 2002, for the first time in the organization's history, voluntary contributions accounted for almost two-thirds of the WHO's overall budget (Yamey 2002c).

Particularly in relation to the WHO's global health security mandate though, not all the newfound trust and confidence in the WHO can be attributed to Brundtland and her initiatives alone. In fact, the trust that member states displayed in the WHO's management of the SARS outbreak in 2003 can arguably be traced to a range of reforms that were initiated as early as 1995 with the decision to revise the IHR. Although Brundtland is reported to have demonstrated a strong commitment to revising the IHR in the last year of her tenure, at the commencement of her term Brundtland was reportedly unaware of the legislation and had to be convinced of its significance by her staff (Kamradt-Scott 2010). Thus the WHO secretariat can be attributed with at least an equal measure of credit for the trust and confidence exhibited by member states in the IO's global health security credentials.

Prior to Dr Brundtland's election as director-general, the WHO secretariat had established the Emerging and Other Communicable Diseases (EMC) unit in 1995 (Weir 2015). The creation of this particular unit, which was later renamed the Communicable Disease Surveillance and Response Unit (CSR) in 1997, had been in direct response to the WHA's passage of two resolutions some five months earlier: *WHA48.7 Revision and updating of the International Health Regulations* and *WHA48.13 Communicable disease prevention and control: new, emerging, and re-emerging infectious diseases* – (WHO 2006a, Weir 2015). As explored more fully in the next chapter, the WHA had passed these resolutions in large part prompted by an increased awareness of the menace posed by biological agents and by emerging and re-emerging infectious diseases combined with the recognized inability of global institutions (including the WHO) to respond effectively to these hazards (Davies 2008). In attempting to redress this recognized shortfall, the guiding vision of the new EMC/CSR unit as outlined by its then-director, Dr David Heymann, was to ensure 'a world on the alert and able to detect and respond to international infectious disease events of international importance within 24 hours' (Heymann 2009). Making full use of the latitude provided by the WHA resolutions, the guiding ethos of the new unit also aimed to 'operationalize' a novel method of working prior to formalizing any innovative developments within elements of the IO's delegation contract such as the revised IHR. What this meant in practical terms was that the team possessed considerable autonomy to experiment with developing novel procedures and policies, and the unit's team began to experiment with a series of changes in how the organization detected, verified, and responded to disease outbreaks (see Chapter Four; see also Davies et al. 2015). In approaching the task this way, the team led by Heymann made a strategic decision to establish new customary IO practice that would then provide the evidence for revising the WHO's health-for-security delegation contract with its principals. As further expanded upon in the next chapter, this 'do first, legislate later' approach understandably consumed the bulk of the unit's time and attention, but it was an approach that the epistemic community was committed to. The most revolutionary change enacted by Heymann and his team at this time was the adoption of a new outbreak verification strategy.

Outbreak verification diverged from the WHO's classical approach to managing infectious diseases in one very distinctive way, notably by using non-governmental sources of information as a basis to identify new disease outbreaks. By 1995 the WHO was receiving literally hundreds of reports about disease outbreaks from international media, NGOs, national laboratories, and collaborating centres, and even other intergovernmental organizations (Grein et al. 2000). Yet under the IO's classical approach towards disease outbreaks, the WHO was prevented from acting on these reports until official notification had been received from the affected member state. In accordance with the novel strategy being utilized by Heymann and his team, however, this had begun to change as the IO became increasingly proactive in response to notifications. As a direct consequence, the numerous pitfalls associated with relying on official government reports, which regularly failed to eventuate or were habitually late, rapidly began to dissipate (Fidler 1999).

In adopting this new strategy the EMC/CSR (and by default the WHO) began to demonstrate that it could use the non-governmental reports effectively and circumspectly. The way the strategy unfolded was that upon receipt of an unofficial report the secretariat would confidentially approach the member state(s) where an outbreak of disease had been reported and seek verification from the government(s) concerned. Where verification was obtained, the WHO was able to respond more rapidly in offering technical assistance and alerting the international community to the presence of the outbreak. Where it was confirmed, however, that no outbreak existed, the WHO was able to assist governments in dispelling potentially harmful rumours that could negatively affect tourism and trade. The new strategy thereby provided a mutually beneficial situation for both member states and the WHO (WHO 2000a).

The adoption of the outbreak verification strategy also corresponded with a number of other related developments though as well. Notably, in 1993 under a joint initiative with UNICEF, the WHO established HealthMapper – a computer software application that enables the IO, governments, and local health authorities to track and map outbreaks of disease (WHO 2000b). The programme, which had been initially developed for the purpose of eradicating guinea worm, was soon revealed to have wider utility. As new geographical information system (GIS) software was subsequently developed throughout the 1990s, the WHO also began to use HealthMapper to track and control a variety of other communicable disease threats as well (WHO 2007b). Further augmenting these initiatives, the International Society for Infectious Diseases had established a global email alert system (Pro-MED) whereby members – several of which were WHO personnel – could freely circulate news about potential outbreaks (Castillo-Salgado 2010); and in 1998 Health Canada, in collaboration with the WHO, developed the Global Public Health Information Network (GPHIN) (Mykhalovskiy and Weir 2006; see also Davies 2015). This latter network functioned as a web-based search engine, continuously scanning some 600 electronic media sources for reports of outbreaks of disease (Grein et al. 2000, p. 99). When a suspected outbreak was identified via one of these sources, the WHO would be alerted. Then, in conjunction with the new outbreak verification strategy, the organization would approach the member state concerned to corroborate or disprove the report.

By July 1999 some 246 disease outbreak reports of international concern had been investigated through using the new systems established by the WHO secretariat and its partners. Of these, approximately 71 per cent of reports had been obtained through non-governmental sources (ibid., p. 100). Although explicit approval of the outbreak verification strategy had not yet been obtained from the WHA, the secretariat demonstrated that it could use such information prudently. Consequently, while it diverged substantially from the IO's classical, established method of working, not one government reportedly expressed any reservation about the new strategy or its corresponding system (Heymann 2005). By early 2000 support for the WHO's new method had grown to such an extent that the decision was taken to formalize and consolidate these developments. The Global Outbreak Alert and Response Network (GOARN) was established in April 2000 (WHO 2000c), and its operation was endorsed by the WHA following the adoption of resolution *WHA54.14 Global health security: epidemic alert and response* in May 2001.

In terms of the WHO's transition from health-for-security to the health-as-security delegation contract, the WHA's ratification of WHA54.14 was a watershed event. In the international context the phrase 'health security' had initially appeared in a 1994 report produced by the United Nations Development Programme (UNDP), which advocated that in the wake of the end of the Cold War a new frame of reference was required – one that moved away from state-centric views of security to a more human-centred approach (UNDP 1994). The UNDP human security report highlighted the menace of infectious diseases as just one area of health security, but this particular 'threat' resonated with a wider narrative that was gaining increasing prominence within a number of high-income countries concerned over the appearance of new diseases like HIV/AIDS and the re-emergence of infectious diseases previously assumed vanquished. As Weir (2015) has recorded, between April 1994 and January 1995 the WHO hosted a series of meetings to discuss the 'threat' of emerging infectious diseases that culminated in the adoption of the earlier resolution *WHA48.13 Communicable disease prevention and control: new, emerging, and re-emerging infectious diseases.* Yet whereas the WHO as the IO tasked with leading and directing international health work might have been expected to grasp this opportunity to immediately re-cast its mandate and thereby reinvigorate its then-tarnished reputation, the wider secretariat demurred for several years. As discussed in the next chapter, a number of explanations can be offered for why this delay transpired, including a range of internal factors such as the transition from one director-general to another and the focus of the CSR team on establishing GOARN; but by late 2000 the WHO secretariat had decided to embrace the health-as-security concept and actively work towards reframing its public health mandate and health-for-security delegation contract. As Guénaël Rodier (2009), who assumed the role of director of the WHO CSR department between 2000 and 2005 later noted:

> The World Health Assembly resolution on global health security, epidemic alert and response, was a milestone firstly because we introduced the concept of global health security for the first time. It was the first time the WHO formally used that term. And it was also a milestone because the World Health Assembly, or member states, formally endorsed what we were doing.

As outlined in the resolution, global health security was narrowly defined by the secretariat to relate explicitly to biological agents, epidemics, and 'communicable disease threats and emergencies' (WHO 2001a). This narrow definition, which at the time gained universal support amongst the IO's principals,[1] should perhaps not be surprising given that it strongly echoed the focus and concern of many high-income countries, several of which had already securitized health within their respective foreign policy frameworks (Davies 2008). The corresponding outcome, however, as Weir (2015, p. 21) observes, was that 'Its title rendered "global health security" equivalent to "epidemic alert and response"'. Over the next few years, several prominent members of the IO's secretariat – and particularly the now-renamed CSR team – embarked on a concerted campaign via the publication of WHO reports and academic papers in prestigious international journals to argue that the IO was the most appropriate mechanism to assist governments in achieving global health security (see, for example, Heymann 2002, 2003, WHO 2003a). Within these documents, the concept of global health security and the WHO's role in facilitating its attainment was presented uncritically as logical, clear-cut, and a rational progression of the IO's health-for-security delegation contract. In effect, the secretariat was engaging in 'securitizing moves' consistent with the Copenhagen School's theory of securitization, but as evidenced by the fact that resolution WHA54.14 had already been adopted with virtually unanimous support and almost no prior warning of the use of this new terminology,[2] the case for the WHO to utilize this discursive tool had already been convincingly made. Said another way, the securitization of the WHO's public health mandate and the move away from its classical 'health-for-security' to a new 'health-as-security' delegation contract had largely been successfully achieved with minimal rhetorical effort from the IO's bureaucratic arm; rather, as explored more fully in the next chapter, it had been the actions undertaken by a concerted group of like-minded individuals at a practical level that proved decisive.

Between April 2000 and March 2003 WHO's reputation for effectively managing what was now being openly described as 'global health security' continued to grow and intensify. The successful operation of GOARN and its partners attracted strong support not only amongst developing countries habitually affected by disease outbreaks, but (especially following the September 2001 anthrax attacks in the United States) the 'network of networks' had also obtained widespread appeal amongst developed countries concerned about bioterrorist attacks (Heymann 2002). With virtually unfettered access to almost every country worldwide and a wealth of international technical expertise to draw upon, GOARN confirmed that the WHO was in a unique position to coordinate global health security – a point keenly promoted by the WHO secretariat (Davies 2008). Hence when the SARS-associated coronavirus did begin to spread internationally in March 2003, the WHO had already proven itself capable of effectively and competently managing disease outbreaks via customary IO practice, even though the formal revision of the IHR – and by default, the IO's health-for-security delegation contract – remained incomplete.

As can be discerned from the above, the actions of Heymann's team throughout this period typified Haas' (1990) typology of IO learning in that a small dedicated group of individuals (epistemic community) actively sought to form alliances with key stakeholders – in this instance, the organization's proximal principals – to advance their own agenda. Having said this, it is important to recall that the health-as-security agenda had also gained considerable traction amongst the IO's member states even prior to 1995 and the passage of resolutions WHA48.7, WHA48.13, and WHA54.14. Accordingly, it would be somewhat disingenuous to label the WHO's explicit adoption of the health-as-security/global health security agenda as a clear example of agency slippage, for the immediate epistemic community tasked with giving effect to the IO's health-for-security mandate was arguably also reflecting the interests of the organization's member states. As later chapters go on to explore, although a number of commentators have postulated that the IO's embrace of global health security can be solely attributed to the influence of the WHO's more proximal principals such as the United

States and the members of the European Union (EU), the adoption of WHA54.14 in 2001 was unanimous. At least for a time, therefore, it appears that there was a global consensus on the WHO's new interpretation of its post-war health-for-security mandate – a consensus that was arguably strengthened by the emergence of SARS.

The WHO response to SARS

The emergence of SARS in 2003 as a global threat has been documented in considerable detail elsewhere (Koh et al. 2003, Abraham 2005, Duffin and Sweetman 2006, WHO 2006a). For the purposes of this book, therefore, only the most basic facts need be recollected. It is now known, for instance, that the disease originally emerged from bats and began infecting people in southern China in November 2002. In March 2003 the pathogen spread to Hong Kong from Guangdong province, carried by an unsuspecting doctor who had been treating SARS-affected patients. The doctor, who had travelled to the Special Administrative Region to attend his nephew's wedding and had checked into a local hotel, unwittingly transmitted the virus to a number of other hotel guests, the majority of whom were international travellers. Although the doctor was himself admitted to hospital the next day, where he later died, several of the travellers he infected departed Hong Kong for their respective destinations around the world. Unfortunately, these individuals had contracted a particularly virulent form of the SARS coronavirus that they then carried with them along major airline routes. These 'super-spreaders', as they became known, subsequently infected others who in turn infected yet further people, setting off a chain of infections that eventually spread to 32 areas.

It is in this regard that that international community was confronted by a unique combination of political, social, and epidemiological factors. The factors themselves – such as the emergence of a novel infectious disease, the reluctance of a government (China) to report the initial outbreaks, the mass movement of people along international airline routes, a series of highly infectious individuals (i.e. super-spreaders), and a high infection rate amongst healthcare workers – were not distinctive per se, but the convergence of these factors within the context of one event certainly was. Moreover, due to this somewhat unique combination of factors, the 2003 SARS outbreak presented a series of peculiar challenges that required a well-coordinated global response. Recognizing the common danger that SARS presented, public health experts, governments, and the WHO collectively sought to contain the threat, successfully accomplishing this objective within four months of the pathogen spreading internationally.

In several respects, the WHO's handling of the 2003 SARS outbreak was consistent with its classic disease management approach. For example, the secretariat issued a series of offers to assist member states in controlling their respective outbreaks of the SARS coronavirus. Where those offers of assistance were accepted, the WHO arranged to send teams of experts to assess the adequacy of control measures and recommend improvements. Similarly, the WHO issued a series of guidance documents outlining how transmission of the contagion could be contained and advising on the latest breakthroughs in treating SARS-affected patients. Nevertheless, the WHO secretariat performed three key roles throughout the 2003 SARS outbreak that diverged markedly from the IO's classical disease management approach: real-time epidemic intelligence coordinator; real-time principal policy adviser; and, perhaps most significantly, the role of government assessor and critic.

Real-time epidemic intelligence coordinator

Disease surveillance on a global scale has always been an imprecise and complicated activity for a number of reasons. Surveillance habitually requires, for example, an advanced infrastructure to support the collection and analysis of epidemiological data. Regrettably, in many resource-poor countries that struggle to provide even basic healthcare services, the infrastructure required for disease surveillance is oftentimes inadequate or non-existent (WHO 2000d). Even in countries with the requisite infrastructure, the data gathered can often vary because of differing opinions on what information is necessary and useful. When the information is then collated at the global level it is not uncommon to find that the data lacks consistency, making it difficult to compare and analyse (WHO 2005b, p. 30). Further, global disease surveillance is also highly dependent upon the willingness of governments to report such information – a willingness that has been observed to be occasionally lacking (Delon 1975, pp. 23–24). Perhaps the largest problem for disease surveillance at the global level, however, has been how rapidly the information is collected, interpreted, and put to practical use.

Timing is essential at each stage of outbreak alert and response. Providing accurate epidemiological data in a timely manner is arguably the single most important tool in preventing and/or containing disease outbreaks (WHO 2000d, p. 6). If used correctly, such information can aid, for example, public health officials in preventing a small outbreak from growing into an epidemic, and an epidemic from developing into a pandemic (Heymann and Rodier 1998). Further, raw epidemiological data by itself does not offer knowledge – it must be interpreted and applied in order for coherent and effective public health interventions to be developed (Bhopal 2002). Disease surveillance thereby feeds into a broader process that collectively is referred to as *epidemic intelligence* (Kaiser et al. 2006), and unfortunately, historically the WHO has had a poor record of making such intelligence readily available.

Until the consolidation of more than 100 different networks under the umbrella of GOARN, the WHO's ability to act on epidemiological information in real-time was largely non-existent (WHO 2003a, 2002b). Instead information about disease transmissions, even epidemics, would filter slowly from the local level to the national level, and then (depending upon the sensitivity of the data) would eventually be reported to the WHO. Delays were not uncommon, with the corresponding effect that the organization's capacity to coordinate global response efforts was repeatedly hindered as the guidelines and advice it sought to provide would appear long after the event had been controlled by national health authorities. Following the CSR's adoption of its global outbreak alert strategy in 1997 and the formal launch of GPHIN in 1998, the WHO's ability to collect, analyse, and interpret epidemiological information in real-time noticeably improved. But the WHO secretariat had not been presented with the opportunity to test these new abilities within the context of an international health crisis, that is, until SARS.

The WHO secretariat's role as real-time epidemic intelligence coordinator unfolded in three distinct phases throughout the 2003 SARS outbreak. The first phase began in late November 2002 following an initial report by a Chinese official of an influenza-like disease outbreak with high mortality that was affecting HCW (Heymann and Rodier 2004a, p. 190). With the exception that HCW were being afflicted though, reports of this nature were not unusual for the time of year (WHO 2003b), and as further information was unavailable, the report attracted little attention. In fact, concern was only really raised following a report just four days later, on 27 November 2002, of a potential influenza outbreak in southern China. This report, which had been identified by GPHIN, prompted the WHO to place its Global Influenza Surveillance Network (GISN) on alert. On 10 December 2002 the secretariat then issued a formal request for further information, but it was dismissed by the Chinese authorities (Brookes 2005); as per GOARN's disease outbreak verification policy, no further action was taken.

The second phase of the WHO response began in early February 2003, following a series of news reports by Hong Kong media that an epidemic of atypical pneumonia was occurring across the border in southern China. The WHO responded immediately by issuing a second formal request for information on 10 February 2003 (Heymann and Rodier 2004b, p. 174). The next day the Chinese authorities convened a press conference where they confirmed that an outbreak had taken place involving 305 individuals and five deaths, but stressed that the outbreak was now well under control (WHO 2003c). Respecting the Chinese government's assurances, the WHO responded by closely monitoring the situation for any signs that the outbreak – which was still believed to be influenza-related – was not contained (WHO 2003d). However, over the next two weeks as further reports began to filter in from Hong Kong, Singapore, and Hanoi of hospital staff contracting atypical pneumonia, laboratory tests failed to isolate any known influenza strain (Stöhr 2003a, p. 1730).

The WHO's third, more intensified phase began on 28 February when Carlo Urbani – a WHO epidemiologist working in-country in Vietnam – notified the CSR department in Geneva of his suspicions that a new contagion was responsible. Urbani's warning prompted the secretariat to intensify its epidemiological intelligence gathering. By 11 March the secretariat had obtained irrefutable evidence of a new disease spreading internationally (WHO 2003c), and in response the WHO issued its first global alert the next day (WHO 2003b). By 14 March, however, it was becoming increasingly apparent that a stronger response was needed (Cohen et al. 2003), and so on 15 March 2003 when it was revealed Dr Leong had boarded a plane to Singapore, the secretariat issued a second global alert and set about assembling international expertise to lead the fight against the disease.

Indeed, the establishment of three 'virtual' global networks of health-care practitioners, epidemiologists, microbiologists and virologists, between 17 and 20 March 2003 was arguably one of the most important public health interventions of the SARS outbreak. Using various forms of advanced telecommunications and Internet-based technologies, the WHO brought together a host of research institutions and individuals to work towards identifying the causative agent responsible, recommending effective treatment options and developing tests that would assist in accurately diagnosing suspected or probable SARS cases (WHO 2003e). It is in this regard that the significance of the WHO's ability to inspire and create these three networks cannot be understated. The networks assembled many of the world's leading health professionals who are regularly required to compete for research funding and prestige in a highly competitive international environment. Drawing on the organization's reputation as an independent technical body, the secretariat created a situation without precedent: each group of scientists, clinicians, and epidemiologists posted their research findings on secure SARS-dedicated websites, enabling normally competing research institutes full access to each others' work. Daily teleconferences further augmented the Internet-based approach, permitting rapid comparison of discoveries and experiences and preventing the duplication of research activities (Abraham 2005, pp. 93–95, Brookes 2005, pp. 101–119). The networks thus allowed the WHO to collect, analyse, and disseminate information in real-time while bypassing many of the traditional constraints of relying on governments and government laboratories to forward information at their discretion and in their own time. As a direct result, the secretariat was able to issue timely policy advice and recommendations which helped facilitate the successful containment of the SARS threat on 5 July 2003, just over four months after it had begun to spread internationally.

Real-time principal policy adviser

As per Article 2(k) of the WHO Constitution, the secretariat is authorized to issue guidelines and recommendations on any matter within the scope of its expertise. Since the IO's inception, therefore, the issuance of temporary and standing recommendations, technical advice, and guidelines has existed as a function that the WHO has regularly performed. In fact, as the WHO was created as a specialized technical agency with the view to it being the highest authority in the field of international public health, the founding member states attached considerable importance to the organization's capacity to issue recommendations and guidelines (WHO 1948b, p. 18). The guidance offered was intended, in principle, to be independent, devoid of political agendas, and based on sound scientific evidence (Siddiqi 1995, pp. 41–51, Beigbeder 1998, p. xix). To encourage this – and in an additional acknowledgement of the IO's own limited financial resources – the secretariat has regularly sought to build collaborative partnerships with independent research laboratories and centres. Through this extensive network of collaborating centres the WHO has established a reputation for providing objective and sound policy advice. As Burci and Vignes (2004, p. 141) have observed, 'The setting of a wide variety of recommendations and other non-binding standards is without doubt the most prolific and successful normative activity of the Organization'.

Yet despite regularly providing policy advice, rarely has the IO been in the position of being able to serve as the principal or leading policy adviser. Instead, as observed in the cases of smallpox and TB, more often than not the WHO's standard approach has been to consolidate the policies and practices that member states have already previously engaged, analyse that information, and then release best-practice guidelines that governments and health authorities may choose to adopt at their discretion. The WHO's guidance, while attracting special status due to its position as a technical agency with independent expertise, is therefore rarely timely due to the processes involved. It is also in this sense that the IO's guidance can usually hardly be described as original.

In the context of the 2003 SARS outbreak, the WHO secretariat issued a number of policy recommendations and technical guidance literally in the midst of a global emergency. The majority of this advice was warmly received by member states and implemented without hesitation, as it was based on established disease control practices such as isolation and quarantine (WHO 2003d). Aided as it was by the three interlinked virtual networks of epidemiologists, clinicians, and scientists, the WHO was also able to issue guidelines and recommendations – in real-time – in several key areas, such as how to conduct SARS-specific disease surveillance; how to build capacity to prevent human-to-human transmission; and importantly, how to treat suspected or probable SARS patients (Heymann 2004, p. 1128).

For example, following the report of Dr Leong – who was suspected of carrying SARS – flying from New York to Singapore, the WHO issued its second global alert on 15 March 2003, recommending that all travellers be screened for signs of infection (Heymann and Rodier 2004a, p. 191). Reacting to the IO's counsel, governments and international airlines began to issue health questionnaires and conduct temperature monitoring of travellers to detect possible carriers of the new disease. Even those governments who had not recorded a single case of SARS within their territory were expected to comply with the organization's recommendations as a minimum precautionary measure (WHO 2003f). While the severity and type of methods used to screen travellers initially varied quite significantly, as the outbreak progressed and the WHO released more information on what methods were proving effective in detecting suspected SARS cases, the tactics employed by these actors became increasingly homogenized (Bell and WHO SARS Working Group 2004). In a few isolated instances, governments were even observed to share highly sensitive infrared technology that had been developed for military applications, adapted to monitor the body temperature of travellers as they entered ports and border crossings, so that the maximum measures recommended by WHO could be implemented by affected territories (Tan 2003). Such offers, ordinarily inconceivable under normal circumstances, served to enhance member states' compliance with the guidelines released by the organization, and many of these measures remained in situ until well after the outbreak was officially declared over on 5 July 2003.

The advice to halt human-to-human transmission issued by the WHO extended beyond the immediacy of the border. As early as 12 March 2003, for example, the WHO recommended that all suspected cases of the new disease should be immediately transported to designated hospitals to be treated, using barrier nursing techniques to limit the risk of transmission (WHO 2003b). Over the weeks that followed, these guidelines were further refined, with the secretariat issuing detailed advice on infection control procedures and the level of personal protective equipment that HCW should use to protect themselves (WHO 2003g). Based on this advice, probable or suspected SARS cases that were identified were usually transported either to the closest healthcare facility or SARS-designated hospital for treatment, or given the choice to enter a period of self-imposed quarantine in their own homes. In this way, human-to-human transmission of the virus was halted in record time as the chain of disease transmission was systematically interrupted wherever it was detected.

Aside from its newfound ability to issue recommendations and policy advice in real-time, one of the more remarkable (and controversial) changes to the WHO's global health security praxis was the decision to target members of the general public with travel advice. The WHO has regularly issued general advice on such issues as vaccination that is readily accessible to international travellers (WHO 2014c). But in the context of SARS, the WHO secretariat intentionally utilized the international media and the Internet to broadcast a range of travel recommendations specifically addressing individuals and their behaviour (WHO 2003h). This was a somewhat controversial decision that attracted criticism from a small number of member states (Cohen et al. 2003), not only as it contrasted with the organization's standard approach of relaying information to the general public via its member states, but principally because in several recommendations the secretariat had recommended that travellers avoid SARS-affected areas (WHO 2003i). Nevertheless, after conferring with the US Centres for Disease Control and Prevention in mid-March 2003 ahead of issuing its advice, the WHO secretariat pursued its controversial policy citing public safety even though such advice was recognized as having potential economic ramifications (Heymann 2005).

Government assessor/critic

The WHO's real-time epidemic intelligence gathering and analysis combined with its principal policy adviser function throughout the 2003 SARS outbreak also culminated in the WHO assuming a very uncommon role, namely that of government assessor. In the heightened uncertainty inspired by SARS' international spread, the IO's recommendations and guidelines attracted elevated status, setting the minimum standards that should be applied to protect populations. Moreover, the WHO – or more precisely, the members of the CSR department – not only began assessing the adequacy of member states' control measures, openness, and transparency, but in a very unusual development the WHO also began to publicly comment on them, and at times even openly criticize member states when they failed to meet the organization's standards. Arguably, by in engaging in such actions the WHO broke the foremost rule of its classical disease management approach, namely that the sovereignty of its member states is sacrosanct. However, in the midst of the global emergency the international community of states failed to contest the IO's actions, potentially establishing a new precedent for the WHO's management of global health security – one based on risk assessment and risk management.

Historically, while measuring performance and producing international standards has existed as an intrinsic part of the WHO's activities, the organization has habitually shunned the role of government assessor. In large part, this has been attributable to the possibility that such assessments may contribute to member states being criticized for their action or inaction on some health-related matter. The WHO bureaucracy's corresponding concern has been that member states may then react by further constraining the IO's authority and autonomy through the imposition of additional control mechanisms (e.g. budgetary restrictions, legal reforms, and similar measures). As Beigbeder (1998, p. 15) has concluded, 'The Organization's authority and the scope of its actions are dependent on the political will of its Member States to grant its own domain and the necessary resources'. As a result, the organization has generally been very careful to avoid engaging in any activity that may jeopardize the goodwill of its member states.

This is not to suggest, however, that recommendations issued by the WHO have never been used as a yardstick to measure member state compliance and/or performance. By their very nature, the production and dissemination of best-practice guidelines encourages comparative analyses to be undertaken. Similarly, the resolutions produced by the WHA or its regional office counterparts have occasionally been used to evaluate the actions or inaction of particular governments (WHO 1998b, pp. 13–14). Yet, in the majority of circumstances, it has been external parties (e.g. individuals, NGOs, the international media, and other member states) that have undertaken such comparisons while the WHO secretariat has stringently avoided making such public evaluations.

In the context of the 2003 SARS outbreak, however, the WHO secretariat assumed the role of government assessor and critic while lacking formalized approval or endorsement by the majority of its member states – a feat it accomplished largely as a consequence of the organization's ability to issue real-time policy advice and recommendations. The uncertainty surrounding the appearance of SARS and how it was spreading caused considerable anxiety internationally. As a result, the WHO's guidelines, recommendations, and advice took on an entirely new level of importance. Indeed, at the height of the SARS crisis the WHO website – where information pertaining to the outbreak was often first released – recorded an average of 10 million hits per day as health professionals, government officials, and concerned members of the public sought to access the WHO's latest advice on SARS (Heymann 2005). Daily press conferences were held for the WHO director-general to report on the latest developments, the content of which was then widely reported by the mainstream print, television, and social media. In short, the IO's recommendations and advice rapidly became viewed as the minimum standards that governments were expected to apply; where such advice was not closely followed, it was not uncommon for the legitimacy of administrations to be openly queried (Loh et al. 2004, Thomson and Yow 2004).

Within this context, perhaps the most blatant example of the WHO assessing the actions and behaviour of its member states pertained to the IO's decision to issue geographically specific travel advisories. In issuing these advisories that warned international travellers to avoid all non-essential travel to SARS-affected areas, the WHO secretariat – and specifically the CSR team – used its own determination to assess member states on how competently they were managing their respective SARS epidemics. Here again the IO engaged in calculated risk assessments based on the epidemiological information it had gathered and the openness and transparency of the member state affected. For example, while Hanoi was cited as an area with local transmission, because Vietnam's government had responded forcefully and rapidly to the threat by quarantining the hospital where the transmissions had been observed to occur, the WHO did not include Hanoi in the travel advisory of 2 April 2003. By way of contrast, because several senior members of the WHO bureaucracy were uncertain about the adequacy of control measures and rate of transmissions occurring throughout southern China, and because the Chinese government continued to decline to fully cooperate with the organization's request to send a team of investigators to the area, the southern Chinese province of Guangdong was among the first to obtain a travel warning (Heymann 2003, Abraham 2005, pp. 96–100).

Intriguingly, not one member state questioned the WHO's authority to issue these travel advisories, even though they did diverge from the IO's standard practices. Instead, the governments of the countries against which travel advisories had been issued were more interested in demonstrating when the advisories were no longer warranted. As Heymann and Rodier (2004a, pp. 193–194) have observed, '[m]eeting these criteria became a strong motivation for governments and populations to collaborate in bringing the outbreaks under control'. To this end, once travel advisories had been issued, the respective governments were observed to fully cooperate with the WHO, sharing information on the number of suspected and probable SARS cases, permitting WHO investigative teams to examine records, assess the adequacy of control measures such as quarantine practices and contact tracing, and to ensure that adequate disease surveillance was being conducted. The investigative teams would correspondingly issue recommendations following their assessment, and it was on the basis of these expert teams' recommendations – not the country's own medical specialists – that the organization would then amend its travel advisory. Moreover, witnessing the WHO's demonstrated capacity to act as government assessor, some governments also invited WHO investigative teams in an attempt to prevent the organization from applying travel advisories. Perhaps the most notable example of this can be observed in relation to the city of Shanghai, China.

Shanghai's status as a special administrative region with consistent economic growth has long been a source of considerable pride for the Chinese government. Thus when SARS cases first began to appear in the city, Chinese officials feared that it too would attract a travel advisory from the WHO and potentially suffer economic losses. To mitigate this possibility, the central government in Beijing issued an invitation to the WHO to send an investigative team to assess the city's surveillance and containment facilities (WHO 2003l). Following the team's investigation, the WHO publicly concluded that Shanghai's health authorities were responding appropriately to the SARS threat, and thus while the organization continued to advocate that all non-essential travel to Guangdong, Beijing, and Shanxi provinces should be avoided, its travel warning was not extended to include Shanghai (Koh et al. 2003, p. 8).

Aside from the organization's rather unusual role as government assessor, arguably the singular, most exceptional aspect of the WHO's response to SARS was its decision to openly criticize the People's Republic of China for attempting to engage in a cover-up. This was a highly uncharacteristic move for an IO that has traditionally shunned even the perception of publicly criticizing its member states. Nevertheless, between April and June 2003 a series of rebukes regarding the Chinese government's actions emerged from within the WHO. In April the organization's chief representative in Beijing, Henk Bekedam, not only criticized China's unwillingness to cooperate fully with the WHO, he also denounced the Chinese health system (and by default its government), stating it had collapsed due to inadequate investment (Ashraf 2003). In May, Peter Cordingley, a WHO spokesperson based at the organization's regional office in Manila, echoed earlier criticisms that Chinese officials had failed to provide adequate information regarding the numbers of SARS transmissions (Parry 2003a). The most pejorative illustration though of the WHO's willingness to criticize China occurred when Director-General Brundtland publicly commented, 'It would have been much better if the Chinese government had been more open in the early stages' (Parry 2003a). In addition, and in an admonishment to the wider international community Brundtland stated, 'I'm saying that as Director-General of the World Health Organization: next time something strange and new comes anywhere in the world, let us come in as quickly as possible' (Crampton 2003).

The impetus for the secretariat's criticisms of the Chinese government appears to have stemmed from two key factors. The first of these was that China's actions in attempting to hide details of the outbreak directly contributed to the spread of the virus, which in turn exposed HCW. It was in this context that the death of Dr Carlo Urbani, the WHO epidemiologist working in Vietnam who alerted the world to the existence of SARS, struck Director-General Brundtland and other senior members of the secretariat particularly hard (WHO 2003k, Brookes 2005). Following Urbani's death, the WHO secretariat issued a series of scathing critiques, increasing the pressure on the Chinese government to permit investigative teams access to the affected areas and fully disclose the extent of the outbreak (Davies 2012).

The second factor prompting the WHO secretariat's criticism of the Chinese government was the fact that the WHO itself began to be publicly criticized. After it was revealed that SARS was likely to have had its origins in southern China and that the Chinese government was actively attempting to deceive the international community regarding the actual numbers of SARS cases, elements of the international media began to criticize the WHO for not publicly condemning China's refusal to fully cooperate (Cohen et al. 2003). The consensus within the organization, which also became publicly disseminated, was that unless the Chinese government was prepared to take all necessary measures to halt the pathogen's spread, the disease would never be eradicated (WHO 2003l). Given that frustration levels were already high within the WHO at the lack of cooperation from the Chinese authorities, when the IO then began to attract criticism for not having publicly spoken out Dr Brundtland took it upon herself to express the WHO's disappointment with China (Abraham 2005, pp. 101–102).

The fact that the Chinese government did not seek to reprimand the WHO secretariat, and Director-General Brundtland in particular, is testament to the authority the IO wielded throughout the SARS crisis. Such open criticism of one of its member states was unparalleled in the WHO's history; and yet, despite being disturbed by the level of criticism it was attracting from an intergovernmental organization, the Chinese government found itself virtually powerless to challenge the secretariat. Moreover, having already suffered such a substantial loss of credibility within the eyes of the international community once, the risk that it may yet attract further criticism prompted a very unusual reaction from China's government in relation to one of the most politically sensitive topics in Chinese relations: Taiwan.

Taiwan's status of representation in international health matters has remained a highly contentious issue ever since its exclusion from the WHO in 1972. When the disputed island territory reported a small number of SARS cases at the beginning of the pandemic, unease amongst the international community began to grow that a diplomatic crisis might also compound the SARS-inspired global emergency. While this unease was temporarily relieved in April 2003 when Taiwanese officials declared (reportedly in testament to its democratic processes) that the outbreak had been rapidly contained (Chen et al. 2003), by early May apprehension had again returned as it was revealed that the island was in the middle of a public health catastrophe. Regrettably, Taiwan's crisis began when officials, in an attempt to conceal an outbreak of SARS and preserve the island's status of success, closed a hospital where new SARS transmissions had occurred. Rather than containing the outbreak, this one action served to disseminate the virus across the entire island as patients were moved to surrounding healthcare facilities to accommodate the hospital's closure. Retracting the earlier assurances that SARS had been contained, the Taiwanese government called upon the WHO for immediate assistance. However, due to the political sensitivity surrounding Taiwan's sovereignty, the WHO was prevented from taking any action except to publicly express, '[w]e are very worried about Taiwan. There are infections in hospital[s], infections in the community, unexplained links. We don't know what's going on there' (Parry 2003a, p. 1055). In response and in what has been considered a 'historic moment', the Chinese government, fearing that if SARS continued to spread unchecked they would attract further international condemnation, permitted a WHO inspection team to visit the island and assist the Taiwanese authorities. The territory subsequently contained its epidemic, and when the WHO removed Taiwan from its 'areas with recent local transmission' list on 5 July 2003, SARS was officially contained.

Conclusion

Collectively, the secretariat's handling of the 2003 SARS outbreak represented a remarkable shift in the IO's more traditional approach to managing infectious disease outbreaks – a shift that admittedly resonated powerfully with the IO's emergent rhetoric of global health security, but, as discussed briefly above, one which also built on the efforts already being taken within the organization to transform its delegation contract. Even before the novel pathogen had emerged particular elements of the WHO secretariat had been actively engaged in a charm offensive, capitalizing on the momentum generated by the passage of resolution WHA54.14 and a wider international consensus that viewed infectious diseases and biological agents as 'threats' to re-cast the IO's public health mandate in security terms. The appearance of SARS and the manner in which some countries responded poignantly highlighted the now evident need for a new way of working. The secretariat's subsequent performance as a real-time epidemic intelligence coordinator, principal policy adviser, and government assessor/critic signalled an organization confident in its ability to manage the risks associated with global health emergencies efficiently and effectively in real-time. It also demonstrated the WHO secretariat could successfully exercise a considerable degree of authority and autonomy in a responsible manner.

Perhaps most significantly, the new roles the secretariat affected in response to the outbreak and member states' behaviour evidenced the value and importance of the global health security agenda and the need to reform the IO's health-for-security delegation contract. Each of the activities executed by the WHO secretariat in coordinating and analysing the epidemic intelligence to provide real-time policy advice, as well as the ability to admonish those governments that were not abiding by expected norms of outbreak transparency, established a new benchmark for the IO's management of infectious diseases. It also revised the parameters of the organization's customary practice, which in turn reinterpreted the IO's health-for-security delegation contract, provided the framework for the WHO's new global health security mandate, and, as explored in the next chapter, gave impetus to finalizing the IHR revision process.

In the wake of SARS, a wide range of diplomats, policy-makers, health professionals, and academics publicly praised the secretariat for its handling of the event, with some even going so far as to hail the IO's actions as having marked 'the point at which a new governance paradigm for global infectious disease threats truly came of age' (Fidler 2004, p. 186). Given such praise and the fact that the organization had handled the SARS outbreak so well, it would be reasonable to assume that should another global health emergency suddenly emerge the WHO secretariat would be well placed to respond in an equivalent manner. In essence, that a new paradigm for maintaining global health security had been established. In order to fully answer this question though, a number of additional factors such as the outcome of the IHR revision process and the WHO's management of both the H5N1 and H1N1 influenza outbreaks require examination. It is to these topics that the rest of the book will now turn.

4
New Powers for a New Age? Revising and Updating the IHR

The WHO's delegation contract with its member states to prevent, control, and ideally eradicate infectious diseases continues to exist as a fluid and malleable one. This is principally because, as noted in Chapter One, the 'contract' – such as it is – is essentially comprised of several provisions and stipulations laid out in a variety of documents, such as WHA resolutions and the WHO's constitutive treaty. Within that array of documents, arguably there is none more important or as comprehensive in outlining member states' obligations and the extent of the WHO's disease eradication powers as the IHR. Originally adopted in 1951, the IHR have continued to form the centrepiece of the WHO's disease eradication health-for-security delegation contract, principally because they represent the only international framework agreement designed to prevent the global spread of infectious disease while minimizing disruption to international trade and travel. Not long after their adoption, however, the IHR came to be viewed as ineffective and insipid, were openly derided, and were frequently ignored. In 1995 the WHO's member states voted to revise and update the IHR. The process subsequently took over 10 years to complete, but following the passage of resolution *WHA58.3 Revision of the International Health Regulations* on 23 May 2005 the revised IHR entered into force on 15 June 2007.

The revised IHR, or the IHR (2005), represent a radically different framework from their predecessor agreements. Scholars and public health officials alike have lauded their adoption (Fidler 2005, Baker and Fidler 2006), and although several significant challenges to their implementation remain (Fischer and Katz 2013, see also Davies et al. 2015), the IHR (2005) have fundamentally altered the terms of the WHO's disease eradication delegation contract with its member states. In fact, as will become clear, the IHR (2005) have been integral to the WHO's efforts to securitize acute health hazards such as infectious diseases. Accordingly, this chapter examines the events surrounding the WHA's 1995 decision to revise and update the IHR, as well as the outcome of that revision process – the IHR (2005) – and its implications for the WHO's global health security mandate. The chapter begins by first examining the terms and scope of the original IHR and surveying the problems that emerged due to member states' non-compliance and obfuscation. Next, the chapter reviews the events that ultimately led to member states' decision to revise and update the framework, the challenges that were then encountered by the WHO secretariat that delayed the completion of this task, and the state of affairs when a new pathogen began to spread internationally in February 2003. The chapter concludes by surveying the outcome of the final phase of the IHR – the Intergovernmental Working Group (IGWG) deliberations – and the import of the new agreement on the WHO's disease eradication responsibilities.

Background to the IHR revision process

As observed in Chapter One, the International Sanitary Regulations were first adopted by the Fourth WHA on 25 May 1951. The WHA's adoption of the framework agreement had long been anticipated, given that the task of developing a universal set of guidelines to prevent the international spread of disease while minimizing disruptions to trade and commerce had been assigned to the Interim Commission of the WHO in 1946. The Commission, which comprised representatives from only 18 governments, initiated a series of preliminary studies but had been unable to make substantial progress in developing new guidelines. As such, in 1948 the newly constituted WHO established the Committee on International Epidemiology and Quarantine to progress with the task, and the committee's first draft was forwarded to the organization's member states for comment in 1950 (WHO 1958). In April 1951, after having reviewed the feedback from member states, a second draft was then developed and an intergovernmental consultation meeting was held – the Special Committee on International Sanitary Regulations – attended by 40 countries (Stowman 1952). The consultation, which lasted for a full five weeks and concluded with the commencement of the Fourth WHA, eventually settled on a negotiated framework agreement that was then submitted to the WHA for review and approval. Following the WHA's endorsement, governments were granted a grace period in which to formally lodge any concerns or objections (otherwise referred to as 'reservations'). Some 21 countries availed themselves of this option, registering a total of 73 items, but most were rejected or withdrawn by the Fifth WHA in 1952, and the new ISR officially entered into force on 1 October 1952 (Edelman 1963).

Reflecting the scope of the largely pan-European agreements that had been drawn up under the International Sanitary Conferences of the late 19th century, the ISR had initially pertained to six 'notifiable' diseases: typhus, cholera, plague, yellow fever, smallpox, and relapsing fever. While these diseases were not the only diseases afflicting humanity, they were recognized as particularly disruptive to international trade and thus were deemed important to circumvent potential conflict arising. Accordingly, member states were expected to notify the WHO of any cases within their respective territories while also taking a series of health and border control measures to prevent the importation of further cases. As Frank Gutteridge (1963, p. 2), former Chief of the WHO legal office, observed, the adoption of the ISR reflected the view that the 'concept of quarantine should be abandoned and instead, by the strengthening and development of national health services and the creation of an improved attitude to health on the part of the general public, the international transmission of disease would be circumscribed or prevented'. Importantly, however, to avoid unnecessary disruption to international trade and travel, the measures that countries adopted were not to be excessive. The ISR thereby set the prescribed benchmark, outlining the maximum allowable measures that countries could take to protect their territory; and in 1955, 1956, 1960, and 1963 small adjustments were made to the regulations to ensure the prescribed measures reflected the best scientific knowledge and practice. Even so, as one external commentator noted:

> Each revision was obsolete on the very day it was published. The changes were natural administrative adjustments to developments in science, but efforts to modernize had always met with embittered bargaining and opposition from those who persisted in holding to the concepts of the past and who thus kept the regulations lagging behind medical development and travel technology. (Velimirovic 1976, p. 478)

In 1969, the ISR underwent their first major revision. Following a similar process to their initial adoption, the (now renamed) Expert Committee on International Quarantine circulated a revised version of the regulations for member states' comments in 1967. The amended draft was adopted at the 22nd WHA in 1969. The most notable and widely recognized change was that the ISR were renamed the 'International Health Regulations', but the more substantive adjustment was in fact the removal of two diseases – typhus and relapsing fever – from the list of notifiable diseases. Both of these diseases had been effectively eliminated in Europe and North America by the late 1940s, but had been included in the 1951 version of the IHR because isolated cases were still reported in Africa and parts of Asia (WHO 1958, pp. 270–271). By 1967, however, many parts of the world were free from these diseases, and while it was recognized that their elimination was not yet universal, in a stunning admission of how inane the regulations had already become the decision was taken to excise the diseases from the IHR on the basis that the areas affected by typhus and relapsing fever frequently declined to report cases when they did occur (WHO 2008a, p. 176).

In 1981, the IHR underwent their second major revision following confirmation of the successful global eradication of smallpox. While justified, the removal of yet another disease from the IHR further underscored the overall lack of regard and relevance with which the regulations were held. Indeed, at no point were calls made to strengthen the IHR, either by creating stronger enforcement mechanisms or by expanding their scope to include other diseases well known to cause considerable human suffering and death (e.g. polio). Similarly, the emergence of several new diseases such as Ebola Virus Disease (EVD), HIV/AIDS, hepatitis C, hepatitis E, as well as the increasing prevalence of recently discovered diseases like Legionnaires' disease and dengue haemorrhagic fever in the late 1970s and early 1980s (WHO 1996a, pp. 15–16, 2011a, pp. 272–273), failed to prompt any re-examination of the IHR as a tool to prevent their spread. As the WHO itself acknowledged:

> The number of outbreaks of communicable diseases has been increasing in recent years. There may be several reasons for this: the increased rapidity of national and international travel and the greater distances travelled; extensive deforestation and irrigation works; neglect of insect and rodent vector control programmes; explosive urbanization and overcrowding associated with poor sanitary conditions; more frequent opportunities for collective gatherings resulting, for example, from improvements in public transport; frequent movements of populations and refugees; social or recreational events; tourism; and large-scale industrial food processing. (Brès 1986, p. 1)

In part, the lack of attention accorded to revising the IHR may be explained by the fact that the WHO had become preoccupied with other initiatives such as the Primary Health Care movement and how to successfully implement the 'Health For All By the Year 2000' agenda while the world was experiencing a global financial crisis (WHO 2011a, pp. vii–viii, Chorev 2012). Yet, arguably, the lack of interest in amending the framework had more to do with how the regulations were generally viewed by the organization's member states, which was far from positive. Much of the damage to the IHR's reputation had to do with the fact that countries habitually ignored their responsibilities, not only in reporting disease outbreaks but also in complying with the maximum allowable measures – a point acknowledged by the WHO secretariat as early as 1975:

> Instances of excessive and useless measures have been numerous in the history of the application of the Regulations since 1951. Apart from unjustified vaccination requirements, which have increased enormously during certain periods of crisis on the pretext of preventing the importation of a disease, we have seen frontiers closed both for travellers and for goods, and international transport by air, rail or road suspended; passengers have been subjected to every kind of victimization and forced by certain administrations to stay at frontier posts for indefinite periods in particularly rough conditions. Unfortunately such measures, while greatly handicapping the movement of travellers and international trade, have not prevented infection spreading between countries. (Delon 1975, p. 24)

Analogous observations were also made by a variety of external commentators. As Carter (1982, p. 111) notes:

> The introduction of excessive measures, either trade restrictions or unnecessary requirements for travellers, is the principal barrier to prompt and frank reporting, and unfortunately it is very often the very countries that do not report that tend to be the first to introduce such measures.

Compounding the situation further, countries were periodically observed to either completely ignore their obligation to report disease outbreaks (Velimirovic 1976, p. 388) or to use alternative descriptions to circumvent reporting diseases subject to the IHR (Plotkin et al. 2007, p. 20). Such behaviour, however, undermined the perceived utility of the IHR by highlighting that there were few incentives for individual member states affected by disease outbreaks to comply with the contractual arrangements they had previously collectively negotiated.

This state of affairs persisted until a series of disease-related events in the early 1990s generated a new impetus amongst member states to reinvigorate their delegation contract with the WHO. Firstly, there were several serious outbreaks of infectious disease. These notably included the reappearance of cholera in Latin America in 1991 a decade after it had been eradicated, an outbreak of plague in the Indian city of Surat in 1994 that caused losses of over US$2 billion to the Indian economy, and an outbreak of Ebola in then-named Zaire in 1995. These latter two outbreaks, which occurred very close to the annual WHA meeting, provided contemporary evidence that both the IHR and the WHO's outbreak policies and procedures needed urgent attention. As David Heymann (2009), former Assistant Director-General of Health Security and Environment, recalls:

> The request from the Assembly came because there were two events that really impacted on WHO's ability to respond to the needs of countries. One of those was the Surat plague outbreak and the other was the Kikwit Ebola outbreak in the former Zaire. It was those two events. They jammed the switchboards at WHO and there was really no system to get the information out to where people could find it even though we were already in an electronic era.

Similarly, Guénaël Rodier (2009), who was a member of the WHO team sent to Surat before taking over as director of the WHO CSR department in 2000, noted:

> Following the plague outbreak in India it was very clear that the IHR were obsolete, and then when emerging infections that were not in the IHR but were reportable like Ebola occurred in Kikwit, then it was even more clear that the IHR not only were obsolete but needed to be revised and be able to integrate emerging infections.

Compounding concerns over ordinary disease outbreaks was the discovery in 1991 of substantial stockpiles of biological and chemical weapons in the First Iraq War, which raised the spectre that disease outbreaks may not always be 'natural' (Tucker 1999, pp. 205–206). This was followed in 1992 by the former Soviet Union's admission that it had maintained an offensive biological weapons programme throughout the entire duration of the Cold War – an understandably disconcerting revelation for many. Aside from the risk of the weapons themselves falling into enemy hands, fear also existed that the scientists who had worked on developing these weapons might be recruited to work for terrorist organizations. The Aum Shinrikyo terrorist attack on a Tokyo subway in March 1995 subsequently appeared to confirm that this fear might well be justified, particularly when it was discovered that the group was actively seeking to develop biological weapons at their headquarters (Fidler 2005, Kamradt-Scott 2010). Consequently, as member states assembled in Geneva a few months later in May 1995 to discuss these various threats to human health, a new consensus emerged to revise the IHR that were universally acknowledged as insipid and outdated and to ensure that the WHO's disease outbreak alert and response capabilities were fit for purpose.

At the same time, momentum was building within the WHO secretariat to revise the IHR and thereby reinvigorate the organization's importance to its principals, namely member states. By 1995 the WHO had become mired in controversy, and the organization's relevance was being increasingly and openly questioned as multiple actors challenged the organization's prominence and leadership credentials (Lee 2009). A lack of funds, precipitated by the decision of the 'Geneva Group' of countries to freeze financial contributions over concerns about the politicization of the WHO, also caused internal schisms and divisions (ibid., pp. 38–39). As Fiona Godlee (1994, pp. 1426–1427), an assistant editor with the *British Medical Journal,* summarized at the time:

> In the absence of coherent policy and strategy direction, conflicts within the organisation are rife. Departments fight over territory rather than cooperating, and communication between them is poor. "All communications have to go through heads of divisions and up through the hierarchy," said one programme director. "The result is that the right hand never knows what the left hand is doing." WHO's internal structure reflects these personal infightings, with units being allocated to divisions not on a logical basis but according to who has what.

Adding to the organization's woes and as noted earlier, the creation of UNAIDS in 1996 was seen by many to be due to the WHO's lack of leadership on the issue and the organization's diminishing relevance – a point that had been very publicly confirmed following Jonathan Mann's resignation from the WHO's Global Programme on HIV/AIDS in 1990 (Fee and Parry 2008, pp. 64–65). Accusations of corruption and bribery that surrounded the director-general at the time, Dr Hiroshi Nakajima, combined with his inability to communicate his vision for the organization, added to a poor image amongst member states and the international media (Godlee 1994, 2014). As a result, the WHO secretariat – and especially its director-general – were actively seeking ways to demonstrate their continued relevance (see Davies et al. 2015). Sensing dissatisfaction from some of the organization's more powerful donor (and thus proximal) states regarding the adequacy of the WHO's disease outbreak response and support activities in the wake of the plague and Ebola outbreaks, and their dissatisfaction with the IHR more generally, certain members of the secretariat embraced the opportunity and directly lobbied the director-general to take further action.

These events, which all occurred within a few short years of each other, were largely situated in and around the WHO. Importantly, however, these events also coincided with the emergence of a new geo-political security environment – one no longer dominated by the Cold War between the United States and the former Soviet Union, and one in which a host of new ideas were being advanced about novel 'threats' to national security. In this environment, and as explored in greater depth below, certain key members of the WHO secretariat played an especially active role, capitalizing on material events to drive home the need to revise and update the IHR. This convergence of material and ideational factors permitted the WHO secretariat to exercise a measure of autonomy, exploiting member states' fears about disease 'threats' to successfully argue for strengthening the international organization's powers. Thus, a firm consensus emerged at the 48th WHA that both the existing IHR and the WHO's disease outbreak response strategies required extensive revision. Passing two resolutions to that effect – *WHA48.7 Revision and updating of the International Health Regulations*; and *WHA48.13 Communicable disease prevention and control: new, emerging, and re-emerging infectious diseases* – the WHA requested the director-general to immediately instigate a programme to evaluate and update the IHR framework. To inform this process, the secretariat was also charged with developing effective disease eradication policies and procedures. These new policies and procedures were then to be used as a basis to revise the IHR and update the organization's disease eradication delegation contract.

The IHR revision process begins

Aware that the IHR revision might be a means to placate member states' growing dissatisfaction with the organization, and particularly his performance as director-general, Nakajima actively pursued his new directive. One of his first decisions was to appoint David Heymann as director of the EMC unit in October 1995. Heymann, a medical epidemiologist, gained his reputation working for two years on the WHO SEP in India and 13 years in sub-Saharan Africa with the US CDC. After joining the WHO in 1988 'on loan' from the CDC, Heymann served as chief of research activities in the WHO Programme on AIDS – a position he held until Nakajima appointed him director of the new emerging diseases department in 1995.

Part of Heymann's remit in his new role was to oversee the IHR revision process, and he assembled a small project team to that effect. The team, which comprised three people, was tasked with coordinating the revision process across member states, numbering approximately 185 at the time. As Heymann (2009) recalls:

> The resolution process for the revision began at the time that the director-general put several different parts of WHO together in the emerging infections program. When we set up the emerging infections program, we realised the IHR were a very valuable framework for what we intended to do in global surveillance and response. And so a vision was developed for how we would proceed and that vision was a world on the alert and able to detect and respond to infectious disease events of international importance within 24 hours. That was the vision, understanding that it was very difficult for countries to report infectious diseases because they knew they could be stigmatized and have great economic loss as well as the negative impact on human health. And so the second part of the vision was changing the norms of reporting so that it became expected and respected to report despite the economic consequences that could occur.

Giving further weight to the WHA's request, Nakajima also authorized the creation of an informal consultation group that met in Geneva in December 1995 to 'consider the international response to epidemics and the role of the IHR in the light of the changes in the global health situation and the increase in international travel and whether revision of the IHR would now be appropriate' (WHO 1996b, p. 1). In the opening session Dr Hu Ching-Li, Assistant Director-General of the Emerging and other Communicable Diseases, Surveillance and Control Division, summarized what was the view of many:

> The current version of the IHR . . . present[s] various shortcomings, such as their limited impact, their relative lack of cost-effectiveness, and the fact that some countries fail to report for fear of incurring

economic losses, for instance by harming tourism. The three diseases currently covered are largely of historical interest and may no longer be the right target. (ibid., p. 4)

The consultation group was subsequently divided into two teams tasked with identifying (a) diseases and/or syndromes to be reported to the WHO for their potential for international spread; and (b) parts of the IHR that needed to be modernized (ibid., p. 7). The group's key recommendations – namely that that the object and purpose of the IHR should remain unchanged and that a specific list of diseases should be dispensed with in lieu of a list of clinical syndromes – set the foundation for how the revision process would proceed over the coming years.

Despite what appeared to be a strong start for the revision process, progress between 1995 and 2000 proved painstakingly slow. Much of the delay can be attributed to problems associated with the new syndromic reporting system proposed by the international group of experts. The basic premise was that by requiring five clinical syndromes to be notified to the WHO,[1] two key faults with the former IHR would be eliminated: first, how to rapidly identify new and unknown emerging diseases; and secondly, how to minimize the time delay in reporting that occurred while laboratories sought to identify the causative agent. To counter the other problem that had arisen in 1994 with countries implementing unwarranted trade and travel restrictions against India, the group also proposed that the WHO be empowered to issue directives to member states on what measures were considered acceptable (ibid., pp. 14–15). Yet although these new measures were recommended in 1995, it took until October 1997 and a further five committee meetings before any trial of the syndromic reporting system got underway.

One of the suggested causes for the delay in commencing the trial was the lack of enthusiasm displayed by member states. As Heymann (2009) recounts:

> I believe that delays came because of a lack of feeling the urgency of the revision process among the member states. And I don't think they felt urgency until the SARS outbreak occurred. So we were working with member states trying to increase attention to the revision, publishing occasional documents in the Weekly Epidemiological Record and discussing it at the World Health Assembly. But they really never engaged in earnest until after the SARS outbreak.

Member states' lack of enthusiasm extended to more practical elements as well, with many even declining to participate in free online discussion forums (WHO 2000e, p. 236). Consequently, the syndromic reporting trial failed to generate the expected outcomes and the trial was prematurely terminated in March 1999 after running for only 18 months. As the official report to the WHO's EB later noted, although syndromic reporting was 'valuable within a national system, [it] was not appropriate for use in the context of a regulatory framework, mainly because of difficulties in reporting syndromes in the field test, and because syndromes could not be linked to preset rules for control of spread' (WHO EB 2001, p. 1). Guénaël Rodier (2009), who took control of the IHR revision process immediately following the conclusion of the trial, agrees:

> The syndromic approach was actually a good idea, but unfortunately it did not work in the end. It is still being used today at the national level, but it could not work at the global level primarily because of the amount of background noise that was generated by the various syndromes we were trialling. The WHO just wasn't capable of dealing with such a large volume of background noise coming from numerous countries. What we found was that only the country could really clarify if it's simple background noise or if it's something worth notifying.

Yet while it may be tempting to blame member states or the sensitivity of the data collection, several internal developments within the organization also contributed to delays. Following, for example, Nakajima's announcement in early 1997 that he would not be seeking re-election, attention understandably turned to appointing his successor. After Dr Gro Harlem Brundtland's appointment in 1998 as the new director-general, the IHR revision process was further delayed by an immediate and extensive review of the WHO's programmes. The outcomes from this review were not made public until early 1999, but it was immediately apparent to some within the secretariat – and particularly the epistemic community that had formed around the CSR department – that Brundtland had arrived with very clear ideas of what the organization should be concentrating on, and infectious diseases were not particularly high on her list of priorities. Mike Ryan (2009), who was appointed to lead the operational side of the WHO's outbreak alert and response function recalls:

> I think the organization didn't really see the value of what we were doing in political terms. Within global outbreak and alert and response we could see it, and we did feel our partners appreciated it,

but when I started running global alert and response our core budget was about $20,000. All of our staff were on short term contracts that were between 3 and 11 months duration. The organization was increasingly becoming orientated towards global policy, normative function, and health systems development.

Thus, although a provisional draft of the regulations incorporating syndromic reporting had been circulated to member states in February 1998, following the trial's collapse and Brundtland's appointment the IHR revision project team were effectively back to square one (Rodier 2009).

By way of contrast to the IHR revisions, the creation and expansion of the WHO's disease outbreak alert and response systems continued to grow, and was yielding some very good results. Building on the work of the GPHIN that had been established in 1998 by the Canadian health department in collaboration with the WHO, the CSR team instituted a series of new policies and procedures to rapidly identify and respond to new and emerging disease outbreaks. At the core of this new approach was the CSR team's desire to transform the WHO into an active risk management organization, as Ryan (2009) recalls:

The WHO has a constitutional commitment to emergency management and risk management, and the IHR as one of the founding principles was what brought countries together in the first place . . . then through the 1950s and 60s with the advent of routine immunization, with the Alma-Ata accords of the 1970s, the move into health systems, health promotion, and the protection of population health became the driving force, and the concept of the WHO as an active risk management organization basically disappeared. By the 1990s though, all of a sudden this recognition of infectious diseases as an acute risk to security re-emerged, and there was a re-birth of interest in emerging infectious disease programmes. In our team we utilized the concepts of event management, intelligence verification and risk assessment, and what we proved was that the risk assessment process wasn't totally owned by the country.

In order to appropriately evaluate the risks though, two core elements needed to be addressed: firstly, the ability to identify outbreaks of disease that were of 'international concern'; and secondly, the ability to identify outbreaks as soon as they began, which would, it was hoped, ideally facilitate their containment at source. If both of these conditions could be met, the CSR team would be successful in returning the organization to its original mandate, but with a slight twist – no longer would health be viewed merely as a vehicle for peace, as health itself was now recognized as fundamental to security at both the international and individual levels.

On the first matter - identifying outbreaks of international concern - the syndromic reporting trial had demonstrated to the WHO secretariat that it was incapable of dealing with large volumes of information. At the same time, the secretariat was adamant that it needed to avoid a list of particular diseases, as any list would become quickly outdated as soon as a novel pathogen emerged. To ensure that it was only notified about outbreaks that might pose an international problem, two new members of the CSR team, Johan Giesecke and Sandy Cocksedge, were tasked with refining the concept of a 'public health emergency of international concern' (PHEIC) and developing a set of criteria to assess outbreaks. An initial algorithm and decision tree was created and distributed to member states to field test, and although debate continued on whether a specific list of diseases should be included, both the concept and the means to identify such outbreaks gained widespread support (WHO 2004a).

The second element at the heart of this new way of working was the ability to use unofficial sources of information to identify PHEICs. This rather radical proposal, which was intended to speed up the identification of emerging outbreaks before they spread, attracted resistance. Intriguingly, however, the resistance arose primarily from within the IO. As Rodier (2009) recalls:

> When I started looking at information outside data formally reported by countries it was not very well received within WHO because it was clearly against tradition. But once I came to appreciate that it was only tradition, I realised there was no formal requirement to analyse or deal with only officially reported information. And we never had a problem with countries saying this is not WHO business. I think it is an important point that not one country ever stopped us. The only problem we had at one point was actually our colleagues in the regional office, but outside the WHO we never had problems.

The CSR team persisted despite internal resistance, and through prudent and sensitive handling of unofficial information was able to demonstrate the benefit of employing non-government sources to both member states and the wider secretariat. As noted in the previous chapter, by July 1999 some 246 disease outbreak reports of international concern had been received by the CSR team and investigated, and of these approximately 71 per cent of reports had been obtained through unofficial sources (Grein et al. 2000, p. 100). Thus although the outbreak verification strategy diverged substantially from the WHO's conventional method of using only government notifications – and before explicit approval of the new risk management system had been obtained – not a single member state reportedly expressed reservations about the new approach (Heymann 2009).

Importantly, however, the same could not be said in relation to the informal expert group's other recommendation that the WHO be permitted to issue directives. Sandy Cocksedge (2009), who was a key member of the IHR revision team, recalls:

> Both the World Trade Organization [WTO] and some WHO member states were uncomfortable with using the concept of measuring a disease event against generic parameters of potential international risk, rather than relying on an established list of diseases. Eventually, the WTO (and WHO) members could see the benefit in a 'public health emergency' process, but were adamantly opposed to having WHO issue directives, rather than recommendations, during international disease events.

This reaction, which was not entirely unexpected, reinforced that there were limits to what member states would accept from their agent despite the collectively negotiated delegation contract and the WHO's disease eradication mandate.

By early 2000 support for the WHO's new policies and procedures (with the exception of issuing directives) had grown to such an extent among member states that the decision was taken to formalize and consolidate these developments. Correspondingly, the GOARN was established in April 2000 under the management of Mike Ryan (WHO 2000f, 2007c), and as discussed in the previous chapter, its operation was endorsed by the WHA the following year with the passage of resolution *WHA54.14 Global health security: epidemic alert and response* in May 2001. In passing the resolution, member states expressed their unreserved support for GOARN and the organization's newfound risk management approach to controlling and halting infectious disease outbreaks, 'particularly with regard to epidemiological investigations' (WHO 2001a, p. 2). The resolution thus served to sanction GOARN's operational methods, which included the specific authority to:

(a) send investigative teams to affected member states;
(b) utilize information from non-government sources to identify outbreaks of disease; and
(c) inform all relevant parties about the organization's investigations and research findings (WHO 2000a, pp. 8–10).

But perhaps most importantly the resolution served the dual purpose of signalling that governments trusted the WHO secretariat to act responsibly in executing these duties. In fact, as noted earlier, the resolution was passed with virtually unanimous support, indicating widespread endorsement amongst the IO's proximal and distal principals.

In many respects GOARN was the practical manifestation of the revised IHR, yet it delayed the revision process in two notable ways. Firstly, the network, which included not only member states but IOs, NGOs, and regional technical organizations and laboratories (WHO 2007c), required the involvement of many of WHO's CSR staff to oversee its creation. What limited human and financial resources that had been allocated to the IHR revision process were subsequently diverted to ensure its successful foundation (WHO 2000f, pp. 2–3). Secondly, it was recognized that any outcomes from the operation of the network had to be reflected in the legal framework for international disease control, namely the IHR. Given this, the network had to be permitted to operate for a time in order to incorporate any changes to the WHO's policies and procedures into the revised IHR. As the secretariat reported in February 2001:

> proposals now are being made within the framework of the revision of the International Health Regulations [to] include the use of WHO's global alert and response network as an additional source of information on public health risks of urgent international importance together with reports from countries, and of the decision tree. (WHO 2001c, p. 63)

To facilitate this objective, Rodier (2009) merged the GOARN and IHR revision teams:

> The first thing was just to start fresh and having Max Hardiman's team based with Mike Ryan's team trying to understand the operations and moving away from the old IHR was so important because there were too many old concepts that could not fly in what we were looking to do. We were developing new approaches to deal with

emerging infections, and that really came to the fore in early 2000. We then introduced all the concepts in a relatively fresh text soon after that.

By mid-2001, following the approval of resolution WHA54.14 and the merging of the IHR and GOARN teams, the IHR revision process again began to slowly move forward. Optimistic that the entire procedure would be rapidly drawn to a close, the secretariat set a new deadline of May 2004 for the framework's completion (WHO 2002c, pp. 158–160). A new draft of the IHR was then distributed to member states and the organization began a new round of regional consultations to gauge governments' views (ibid.). Yet despite the initial optimism, progress was again hampered; the events of the 11 September 2001 terrorist attacks, other negotiations such as the failure of the Biological and Toxic Weapons Convention (BWC), the Second Iraq War, and the fight against terrorism more generally, distracted governments and the secretariat alike (Heymann 2009). Indeed, particularly in terms of negotiations it seems elements of the WHO secretariat became preoccupied with the BWC, as Mike Ryan (2009) observes:

> We had people here [within the WHO] who were really pushing for that engagement and there was a lot of tension internally over that because we did not want the IHR to become the proxy replacement for a failed discussion on the verification mechanism for the biological weapons convention, and there was a point where that was really becoming an issue.

As a result of these distractions, by February 2003 when SARS began spreading internationally the process to revise the IHR remained far from complete.

The IHR Intergovernmental Working Group negotiations

The 2003 SARS outbreak and the WHO's prudent management of the event generated significant political interest amongst the IO's member states to conclude the IHR revision process as speedily as possible. In May 2003, at the height of the SARS outbreak, member states passed resolution WHA56.28, observing that SARS had 'given concrete expression' to the challenges the international community confronted in combating infectious diseases, the inadequacy of the existing IHR framework, and the need to conclude the revision process as soon as possible

(WHA56.28, preamble – WHO 2003m). In response, WHO Director-General Brundtland allocated new financial resources and personnel to convene the IHR IGWG. The most intensive phase of the IHR negotiations then officially began in November 2004 with the first of what ultimately became three IGWG meetings.

It was initially believed a two-week round of negotiations would be sufficient to conclude the IHR revisions. To that end, 155 of 195 member states assembled in Geneva on 1 November 2004 to agree on a final version of the framework. Yet, despite the best of intentions and a very formidable chair in the person of Ireland's Ambassador, Mary Whelan, the first IGWG negotiations broke down over several contentious areas. As Whelan (2008, p. 9) later noted:

> My ambition during this first session was to ensure: a first reading of the text to identify problems; a second reading to seek to reconcile differences and move towards consensus; and an outcome document that might serve as the basis for further work. The first objective was achieved, the second partially achieved and, as far as the third objective is concerned, I had been too sanguine.

Aside from the standard diplomatic wrangling and posturing that accompanies any intergovernmental negotiations, two core issues served to delay finalization of the revised IHR framework until the third and final meeting of the IGWG in mid-May 2005.[2] As Rodier (2009) observed:

> The IGWG was interesting because it put the text on the table and then the text started to be challenged from two angles. One angle was national sovereignty. As you know, the IHR today is a result of negotiation between the will for global solidarity, and at the same time, the need to maintain national sovereignty. The second angle I think was the core problem really in that the IHR, because it involves global health security issues, is an area where public health overlaps with national security.

Indeed, both elements – state sovereignty and the health/national security nexus – proved instrumental in (re)shaping the WHO's global health security authority via the IGWG negotiations. It may be recalled, for instance, that the actions of IOs can establish new interpretations of IO authority – a phenomenon accepted under customary international law (see Chapter One). The WHO's management of SARS could have been interpreted, therefore, as having established new forms of IO authority, empowering the WHO to replicate its real-time epidemic intelligence coordinator, principal policy adviser, and government assessor/critic roles that informed the organization's risk management approach for containing outbreaks. Importantly, however, throughout the IGWG meetings several elements of the WHO's new approach to managing global health security were systematically scaled back due to concerns regarding state sovereignty and/or national security.

One of the areas where this was perhaps most clearly demonstrated pertained to the WHO's real-time principal policy adviser role. As discussed in Chapter Three, as the SARS coronavirus began to spread internationally the WHO secretariat issued a number of recommendations that advised travellers to avoid areas affected by the disease. Although the WHO possessed a long history of issuing recommendations on disease outbreaks, the secretariat had never previously addressed them to the general public. Rather, the organization's conventional approach had been to communicate information to its principals (member states), which in turn would advise their citizens as they deemed appropriate. In this regard, the WHO was effectively kept at arms' length from communicating directly to the general public. In the context of SARS, however, the WHO secretariat dispensed with its standard protocol and laid the foundation for its real-time principal policy adviser role to become the new custom. Purportedly at the time no government objected to the IO's actions, but throughout the IGWG meetings member states moved to rein in the WHO secretariat's autonomy in this area in two notable ways.

The first aspect of the WHO secretariat's real-time principal policy adviser role that member states challenged was the IO's ability to independently declare a PHEIC. Whereas in an earlier 2004 draft of the IHR the secretariat had advocated that it would simply 'inform health administrations of the occurrence of a public health emergency of international concern and of the control measures taken by the health administration concerned', as early as the second day of the first IGWG meeting member states were demanding that this be changed (WHO 2004b, p. 9). Correspondingly, the secretariat was forced to accept a different position and, as the negotiations proceeded, it became increasingly apparent that the organization had to make certain guarantees that this power would not be abused. As Whelan (2008, p. 9) recalled:

> to be effective, the IHR had to give to an international entity that was reasonably free from political interference the key role in determining a public health emergency. That entity had to be the

Director-General of the WHO. This was not immediately acceptable to all delegations, although there was no realistic alternative. Given the economic and other consequences that would flow from the exercise of such authority, governments were understandably concerned that there should be adequate consultative mechanisms in place to ensure that this authority was exercised with prudence, and after having taken the broadest possible advice.

Moreover, Whelan (2009) was instrumental in ensuring member states' concerns were addressed:

> That was the one occasion when I felt the secretariat perhaps did not understand fully the concerns of member states. Everybody realised that the determination of a PHEIC had to be vested in the organizational structure of the WHO, but that's a huge burden to put on any organization. So, it was important to have someone in the chair who understood the concerns of governments. In the drafting group before the February meeting, we went through the proposed text paragraph-by-paragraph with various members of the secretariat, the legal office, and the director-general's office so that it represented what I felt governments could accept. So, in that sense, the draft text prepared in advance of the February meeting was not a chair's text per se, but more a text indicating where the chair thought a consensus might be possible. It was always a question of finding the right balance that did not diminish the role of the director-general, while also recognising the concerns of member states.

Various textual amendments were subsequently introduced, scrutinized, adjusted, or rejected, and then evaluated again throughout the course of the three IGWG meetings, all in an attempt to placate member states' concerns regarding the WHO's ability to unilaterally declare a PHEIC. Eventually, these debates culminated in the creation of an entirely new entity – the IHR Emergency Committee – that the director-general is required to convene whenever a suspected or actual PHEIC is underway (see Articles 12, 48, and 49 in WHO 2008b, pp. 14–15, 31–32). Membership of the IHR Emergency Committee is strictly limited to technical experts (nominated by member states), but through the protocols associated with this new committee any member state affected by a potential or actual PHEIC is entitled to present their case prior to any final determination being made on whether a disease event of international concern is occurring. Further, the director-general is obliged to take the views of the affected member state(s) as well as those of the IHR Emergency Committee into account before declaring a PHEIC. This new process, designed by member states and embedded into the revised IHR framework, has thereby been intended to negate the WHO secretariat's previous autonomy of unilaterally declaring a PHEIC.

The second aspect of the WHO's real-time principal policy adviser role to be challenged in the IGWG was the IO's ability to unilaterally issue recommendations. Here member states, again via the mechanism of the IHR Emergency Committee, moved to ensure that a more thorough consultative process would be followed prior to the WHO secretariat issuing recommendations that may be economically or reputationally damaging. Moreover, under the terms that member states agreed upon the WHO secretariat is limited to issuing temporary recommendations on

> health measures to be implemented by the State Party [member state] experiencing the public health emergency of international concern, or by other States Parties regarding persons, baggage, cargo, containers, conveyances, goods and/or postal parcels to prevent or reduce the international spread of disease and avoid unnecessary interference with international traffic. (Article 15 paragraph 2, WHO 2008b, p. 16)

If a strict interpretation of Article 15 is taken, therefore, not only could it be argued that WHO-issued travel advisories are disallowed as they technically are not 'health measures',[3] but also that the WHO secretariat must return to directing all communications (including recommendations) exclusively at member states. In fact, as per Article 49, the director-general is only permitted to share recommendations with the general public after having conveyed such information to member states (see paragraph 6, WHO 2008b, p. 32). While in practice these protocols did not prevent the director-general holding press conferences or from issuing statements (including travel advisories) in the context of the 2009 H1N1 influenza pandemic (see next chapter), it is nevertheless clear that the IO's principals attempted to institute new legislative control measures on their agent via the IHR (2005) to limit autonomy and protect state sovereignty.

In the same way, the consultative process now required under the IHR Emergency Committee effectively seeks to curtail the WHO secretariat's role as government assessor and critic. While under the revised IHR the director-general can conceivably still express reservations about a member state's ability to contain a PHEIC if the country has limited technical capacity in disease outbreak control, equally the requirement for the IHR Emergency Committee to hear the views of an affected member state creates new opportunities for political coercion, whether perceived or actual. As explored in the next chapter, accusations of external political interference assailed the IHR Emergency Committee at its inaugural formation in 2009, prompting a series of internal and external investigations to identify whether the WHO had been unduly influenced into declaring a pandemic. In this context, it is not difficult to appreciate that in future the director-general would proceed even more cautiously before publicly commenting on a government's ability to manage a disease outbreak – an objective that was undoubtedly the intention of the IO's principals throughout the IGWG.

Related to the above, when proposals were put forward in the IGWG to expand the WHO secretariat's role as government assessor, the proposition was met with staunch resistance. It had been suggested, for example, that whenever a potential or actual PHEIC was suspected to be the result of a chemical, biological, radiological, or nuclear (CBRN) event or terrorist incident, member states should be compelled to provide biological samples to the WHO secretariat for verification. Several member states – and one regional arm of the WHO in particular – argued vigorously, however, that granting the secretariat such verification powers would politicize the IO by turning the organization into the 'health police', which was fundamentally at odds with its traditional role of 'WHO-as-physician'. The line of reasoning that was advanced to support this position, which on more than one occasion threatened to derail the negotiations, was primarily two-fold: firstly, that the WHO needed to maintain the image of neutrality to facilitate its more important health work; and secondly, that other IOs such as the International Atomic Energy Agency (IAEA) and/or the UN Security Council were better placed to deal with verifying CBRN incidents. It was contended that if member states were to otherwise grant the WHO secretariat the means to compel governments to provide samples of a causal agent (in order to verify whether a CBRN agent was involved or not), it would not only potentially risk compromising the national security of those member states concerned, but the WHO could additionally become embroiled within matters outside of its traditional public health remit. The regional bloc of member states thereby concluded that by ceding these powers to the IO, member states risked irreparably politicizing the WHO.

Having said this, perhaps one of the most important elements of the WHO's new role as government assessor and critic – the ability to 'name and shame' governments to induce cooperation – has been enshrined by member states in the IHR (2005). Article 10, paragraph 4, of the revised framework stipulates, for instance, that the WHO secretariat is authorized 'when justified by the magnitude of the public health risk' to publicly share all information about a suspected PHEIC whenever a government fails to accept the WHO's assistance (WHO 2008b, p. 13). In the event that member states then impose measures that 'significantly interfere with international traffic' the WHO secretariat is further authorized, as per Article 43, paragraph 3, to publicly disseminate the justification(s) used by these governments (ibid., p. 29). Reflecting the inviolability of state sovereignty, no additional authority has been granted to the WHO secretariat either to intervene in the domestic affairs of a country or enforce compliance with the IHR (2005). Nonetheless, as the 2003 SARS outbreak revealed, the ability to 'name and shame' can be a powerful motivating force with recalcitrant governments. Throughout the IGWG deliberations, China's refusal to be open and transparent about the extent of SARS transmissions served as a persuasive reminder of the need to grant the IO such authority. With this license now embedded in the IHR (2005), the WHO secretariat is empowered to replicate its function as government assessor and critic.

Arguably, however, the single most critical feature of the WHO secretariat's new approach to managing global health security – namely its real-time epidemic intelligence coordinator role – has been strengthened under the revised IHR. This function, which has been preserved under Article 9 of the IHR (2005), clearly states that the WHO secretariat 'may take into account reports from sources other than notifications or consultations and shall assess these reports according to established epidemiological principles' (WHO 2008b, p. 12). The ability to utilize non-government (otherwise described as 'unofficial') sources of information had been previously endorsed by member states under resolution *WHA54.14 Global health security: epidemic alert and response* in May 2001, but its inclusion in the revised IHR legislative framework some four years later further reinforced the WHO secretariat's new delegated authority. It also marked a profound break with the IO's former classical approach to disease eradication that routinely acquiesced unswervingly to state sovereignty even where verified reports to the contrary existed.

Conclusion

The third and final meeting of the IHR IGWG concluded around 3 am on Saturday 14 May 2005, just two days prior to the commencement of the 58th WHA at which the revised framework was to be adopted.

With the exception of the delegation of Cuba, the IHR framework was unanimously approved by the IGWG, and the WHO secretariat then worked throughout the weekend to ensure the final report and all related documentation was translated into the six official languages of the IO for the start of the WHA. Some eight days later, member states of the 58th WHA passed resolution *WHA58.3 Revision of the International Health Regulations* on 23 May 2005, concluding the decade-long IHR revision process and formally endorsing the majority of the WHO secretariat's new approach to managing global health security.

Indeed, despite the fact that the IHR (2005) makes no explicit mention of the phrase 'global health security', it is clear that the revised legislative framework is integral to the WHO's reframing of its public health mandate in security terms. Just two months after the IHR (2005) officially entered into force on 15 June 2007, for example, the director-general released the 2007 World Health Report *A Safer Future* that explicitly outlined the WHO's new global public health security mandate. In announcing the release of the new report, the director-general's efforts were supplemented by other members of the secretariat that sought to explicitly draw links between the revised framework and global health security, highlighting that the IHR (2005) were the only tool to help attain and maintain this goal (Rodier et al. 2007). It was a goal, however, that even in 2005 as member states were meeting in Geneva to endorse the revised IHR, was under threat from a novel strain of influenza in the form of H5N1 'bird flu'.

5
Pandemic Influenza: 'The Most Feared Security Threat'

As government officials met in Geneva at the 58th WHA to endorse the revised IHR (2005), alarm was mounting that the world confronted an imminent new menace. The emergence and progressive spread of the highly lethal H5N1 avian influenza 'Bird Flu' virus from 2004 onwards had captured the international community's attention. It had also directly fed into the 'threat' from the emerging and re-emerging infectious diseases narrative that had been actively promoted since the 1990s – and in the particular case of influenza – that the world was 'overdue' for another pandemic. Ultimately, however, Bird Flu did not become the etiological agent for the first influenza pandemic of the new millennium. Rather, it was another novel strain of H1N1 influenza (A) usually found in pigs that was first identified in a small Mexican village in 2009 that achieved human-to-human transmission and spread around the world.

In the lead up to the 2009 H1N1 influenza pandemic, the WHO had been engaged in a decade-long campaign to highlight the dangers of another influenza pandemic. In a classic securitizing move, this culminated in the organization labelling the disease 'the most feared security threat' in the 2007 World Health Report *A Safer Future* (WHO 2007a, p. 45), elevating the influenza virus above all other disease threats. The focus of this chapter is to examine the WHO's approach to influenza and how this approach has changed and adapted over time. Accordingly, the chapter commences with a brief survey of the WHO's efforts in the 1950s – from its initial scepticism of protective measures to its proclamation that influenza vaccines were the 'cornerstone' of preparedness. Next, the chapter reviews the organization's attempts to embed influenza preparedness within country health systems in order to devolve itself of responsibility, until that is an outbreak of H5N1 avian influenza in 1997 in Hong Kong prompted the WHO to re-evaluate its stance. The chapter then moves to examine how the organization has sought to manage the emergence and progressive spread of the H5N1 virus by securitizing the disease, before exploring the WHO's role in the 2009 H1N1 influenza pandemic and how it has affected its global health security mandate in the wake of the IHR (2005) revision.

First days: the WHO and flu

Public perceptions regarding the menace posed by influenza to international society altered markedly in the wake of the 1918 Spanish Influenza pandemic. The widespread illness and death prompted by this event spurred new research into identifying its cause; as a result, a small team of scientists isolated the virus in 1933 (Smith et al. 1933). It also triggered the desire to regularly monitor outbreaks of 'epidemic influenza' by existing international health organizations such as the OIHP and LNHO (Sydenstricker 1924, Hampton 1925), efforts that were understandably interrupted by the outbreak of WWII. When the decision was taken in 1946 to establish a new universal health organization, one of the first tasks assigned to the Interim Commission of the WHO was to develop a new programme to monitor and study the disease. The World Influenza Centre (WIC) was founded in London the following year with the three-fold objective to: (a) prevent future pandemics, (b) develop control methods to limit impacts arising from a pandemic, and (c) to limit wherever possible the economic consequences of influenza epidemics and pandemics. To complement the WIC and inform the WHO's broader influenza-related activities, in 1950 the Third WHA also approved the creation of an Expert Committee on Influenza (Payne 1953, see also Doull 1948). The Committee met only once in 1952, but the meeting drew together a number of well-respected and highly influential influenza experts (mostly from European countries and the United States) to decide on the methods and structure of a new international scientific research network – the GISN (WHO 1953).

The basic premise of the GISN was to create an international network of research laboratories that would assist the WHO to provide technical support to member states in controlling influenza outbreaks, epidemics, and pandemics. Accordingly, to this day the primary function of the network continues to be the identification and isolation of strains of the virus that are circulating, which it accomplishes by receiving samples from participating countries via National Influenza Centres (NICs).

The NICs forward samples to WHO reference laboratories (otherwise known as WHO Collaborating Centres), where the strains are isolated and categorized. The epidemiological intelligence gathered from these activities is then consolidated and shared with pharmaceutical companies to develop therapeutic countermeasures such as influenza vaccines. In 1952, when the GISN was founded, some 40 laboratories immediately joined the network (Jensen and Hogan 1958), and by 1977 the association had grown to 98 NICs spread through 70 countries (Pereira 1979). Since then, both the number of NICs and reference laboratories has continued to grow, so that at the time of writing the GISN comprises 141 institutions in 111 countries, supported by a total of six WHO Collaborating Centres based in the United Kingdom, the United States, Japan, Australia, and China (WHO 2014d). In 2011, the GISN was renamed the Global Influenza Surveillance and Response System (GISRS) to signify the change from a previously publicly funded technical cooperation system to a public-private partnership following the passage of the 2011 PIP Framework (ibid., Kamradt-Scott 2013).

When the GISN was established in 1952 it was still not apparent how the international community could best protect itself against the disease. Although the virus had been isolated in 1933, it took a number of years before clinical trials to test the efficacy of vaccines were launched. Somewhat intriguingly, the majority of clinical trials were initiated by military forces on account of the outbreak of WWII and due to concerns that there would be a repeat of the 1918 Spanish Influenza pandemic at the end of the second global conflict (Francis 1947). Once the war had concluded though, responsibility for developing pharmaceutical countermeasures once again passed into civilian hands; yet by 1952 results from trials conducted in the United Kingdom, the United States, and elsewhere were still inconclusive. As a result, the WHO Expert Committee on Influenza was forced to conclude in its first (and only) report that:

> Experience in the past has shown that it is possible to reduce the incidence of influenza by means of immunization. Nevertheless, influenza virus vaccination is still, in the opinion of the committee, an experimental procedure, since success or failure is determined by a number of different factors which demand further experimentation. (WHO 1953, p. 10)

Undeterred, work on vaccines continued apace, and with the commencement of the 1957 'Asian Flu' pandemic questions over the efficacy of influenza vaccines were firmly resolved. In fact, as a direct consequence of countries' widespread use of vaccines throughout the 1957 pandemic, the WHO Expert Committee on Respiratory Virus Diseases (which succeeded the Expert Committee on Influenza) proclaimed, 'Experience in many countries has now established vaccination as the most efficient method for the prevention of influenza' (WHO 1959b, p. 15). This modification of views was due, in large part, to the considerable evidence that had been collated from annual seasonal influenza epidemics and various clinical trials (Davenport 1979). Added to this, the information obtained from the widespread use of laboratory-based influenza surveillance and community-based public health surveillance in the context of the 1957 Asian Flu pandemic further strengthened the case for vaccines and validated the importance of both the WIC and the GISN. As Jensen and Hogan (1958, p. 140) noted, 'The role of the laboratory in defining and following the spread of an infectious agent has never been more dramatically shown than in the present epidemic of Asian influenza'. These techniques allowed national health authorities (and by default the WHO secretariat) to not only monitor the progressive spread of the 1957 pandemic, but also to identify and isolate the strains of virus responsible, distinguish between 'influenza-like illnesses' and the number of real cases, develop strain-specific vaccines, and then assess their efficacy (Stewart 1958, Roden 1963).

It is in this regard that the late 1950s marked a particular turning point in the development of influenza prevention and control practices. The experience of the 1957 Asian Flu pandemic cemented the importance of vaccination as an effective strategy to reduce human morbidity and mortality (Kamradt-Scott 2012). As a result, over the next decade emphasis was increasingly placed on refining the vaccines to ensure better efficacy, less toxicity, and greater yield within a shorter timeframe. The WHO secretariat's actions throughout the 1957 pandemic (and the subsequent 1968 'Hong Kong Flu' pandemic) in consolidating epidemiological intelligence, providing policy advice, and encouraging governments to develop national surveillance programmes and pharmaceutical manufacturing capacity was consistent with the organization's classical approach to managing global health security. It also contributed to the WHO global influenza programme being perceived as 'an authoritative source of information on the occurrence of influenza and its spread from one country to another' (WHO 1969b, p. 8).

Perversely, however, the proven benefit of surveillance techniques and the efficacy of influenza vaccines had a deleterious impact on the WHO's global influenza programme. Moreover, the WHO secretariat was somewhat complicit in this de-escalation. As early as 1959, for example, the WHO Expert Committee on Respiratory Virus Diseases officially recommended that:

> the laboratory network originally organized under the programme should be brought into closer relationship with national public health authorities. This is necessary for two reasons – first, in order that the influenza centre of the country may be alerted to, and may organize the investigation of, outbreaks in distant parts of the country, of which it might otherwise not learn in time, and secondly so that the centre may keep the health authorities informed of the appearance of unusual viruses or epidemics elsewhere in the world and of the appropriate technical measures which should be taken. (WHO 1959b, p. 22)

The report – and by default, the WHO secretariat – thereby advocated that member states take greater carriage of influenza programmes, embedding them within existing national public health structures. When this advice was also viewed in light of the success of vaccines (which could be produced by state-owned or government-sponsored pharmaceutical manufacturers), it gave additional weight to the notion that influenza was a largely controllable disease that could be managed effectively by individual governments.

Accordingly, the perception emerged that there was less need for international resources – a perception that the WHO secretariat failed to dissuade its principals from holding in what might be described as an example of agency shirking. Noting the downturn of interest, for example, in 1988 the then-directors of the WHO Collaborating Centres issued a statement calling for the WHO influenza programme to be 'maintained and strengthened because, by facilitating the earliest possible detection of new epidemic strains of influenza virus and recommending the use of new antigenic variants for vaccines, it provides the foundation for activities to prevent and control the disease' (WHO 1988, p. 457). The call went largely unheeded though, and was not repeated. As a result, even as the 'threat' of emerging and re-emerging infectious diseases was gaining political attention throughout the mid-1990s (Lederberg 1996), and notable virologists were warning the world was 'overdue' for another influenza pandemic (Webster 1994, Webster and Kawaoka 1994), by 1996 the number of WHO personnel overseeing the organization's influenza work had been reduced to one staff member (Kamradt-Scott 2012).

In many respects, the WHO secretariat's actions throughout this period exemplified the organization's classical approach to managing infectious diseases. For instance, the WHO secretariat limited its activities to coordinating influenza-related epidemiological intelligence, which it accomplished via oversight of a network comprised exclusively of externally operated (and externally funded) laboratories and institutes. The second function that the WHO performed was that of providing policy advice, realized through the periodic gathering of internationally recognized influenza experts. Reflecting the post-MEP aversion to directing member states and evaluating their performance (or lack thereof), the WHO declined to scrutinize whether governments had in fact followed its recommendations in developing surveillance systems and pharmaceutical manufacturing capacity. Member states were instead encouraged to 'do the right thing', which – while the GISN did continue to grow and expand – meant that influenza failed to be prioritized.

For the purposes of this book, it is equally important to note that throughout this entire period the WHO did not seek to securitize the disease. Within the broader health community periodic references were made to the 1918 Spanish influenza pandemic and the 'threat' of an equivalent epidemiological event (Walters 1978, Pyhälä 1980), but these comments were usually made within the context of debates surrounding public health expenditure in an attempt to heighten awareness and/or obtain additional resources for influenza. Even in this respect, the WHO secretariat generally refrained from such advocacy work, preferring instead to publish technical advice in the *Weekly Epidemiological Record* to be 'widely distributed to health authorities, influenza centres, and other interested institutions and persons' (Ghendon 1991, p. 513). In this regard, the organization's global influenza programme was explicitly public health-focused, emphasizing traditional, proven biomedical techniques, methods, and interventions. Equally, however, within this environment influenza-as-a-public-health-priority languished, so much so that the WHO's own programme was severely curtailed.

The emergence of H5N1 and the WHO's securitization of flu

Political interest in the WHO's influenza programme only really re-emerged in 1997, following an outbreak of H5N1 avian influenza in Hong Kong that killed six out of 18 infected people (Snacken et al. 1999). While small in terms of overall human morbidity and mortality, the outbreak caused significant international anxiety that a new pandemic was imminent. As a result, Hong Kong's health minister, Margaret Chan, controversially ordered the destruction of the territory's entire poultry population on the grounds that it was the most appropriate action to take – a decision that was reportedly based on the epidemiological evidence (Shuchman 2007). The subsequent medical consensus that emerged was that Chan's actions likely prevented a new pandemic (MacPhail 2009), but the outbreak renewed international pressure on the WHO to reinvigorate its influenza programme, and the organization immediately began developing new policy guidelines on how its member states should prepare for mitigating an influenza pandemic. The WHO's first official pandemic influenza preparedness guideline document was then released in 1999, and outlined in broad terms the steps that countries should take to protect their respective populations from the 'pandemic threat' by developing vaccination and other control strategies, strengthening surveillance systems, and ensuring access to critical supplies such as vaccines and personal protective equipment (WHO 1999b).

Yet between the mid-1990s and late 2003, high-level political interest in influenza prevention and control continued to fluctuate. In the lead up to and the subsequent creation of the MDGs, much of the world's public health community had become preoccupied with engaging the political elite about other infectious diseases (such as HIV/AIDS, malaria, and, to a lesser extent, TB) and health objectives such as improving maternal and child health. Within this milieu, and as reflected in the 1998 World Health Report summary document, the WHO influenza programme struggled for prominence (see WHO 1998c, pp. 9–12). In the technical sphere, prominent scientists, epidemiologists, and medical professionals did continue to progress matters, establishing new web-based surveillance tools such as FluNet and publishing journal articles, commentaries, and opinion pieces warning of the dangers of a new influenza pandemic (Flahault et al. 1998, Dowdle 1999, Fauci 2003). Yet progress remained slow. In 2001, in an attempt to 'raise the profile of influenza as a disease that has significant *economic as well as public health* consequences throughout the world', the WHO secretariat issued a call for proposals to develop a 'Global Agenda on Influenza Surveillance and Control' (Stöhr 2003b, p. 1744, emphasis added). The Agenda was launched the following year and identified four key goals:

- Provide impartial guidance to all parties on priorities for research and development and national/global action for influenza control;
- Support coordination of action for influenza control and surveillance;
- Support implementation of identified priorities; and
- Support advocacy and fundraising. (ibid.)

A further 17 priority activities were identified under these key goals, such as increasing vaccine usage, enhancing surveillance, standardized training, assisting with national and regional pandemic planning, and so on (ibid., pp. 1746–1748). Giving effect to these new priorities, the WHO secretariat released the first draft of the *Guidelines on Vaccine and Antiviral Use during Influenza Pandemics* in October 2002 and held its first influenza surveillance and epidemiology training course the following month (ibid., p. 1745). Proposals were also advanced for the creation of a new influenza advisory group to inform the organization's activities and forums (ibid.).

Importantly, however, there again appeared to be little urgency to the WHO secretariat's efforts. Several internal and external factors can conceivably account for this. First, as discussed in the previous chapter, during this period the WHO secretariat – and specifically the CSR department – was engaged in revising and updating the IHR, evaluating the results of the syndromic reporting trial, and establishing the GOARN. Given the limited number of CSR personnel, it can be reasonably assumed that these activities occupied the majority of their resources and time. Individual diseases that were not currently active (like pandemic influenza) were simply not viewed as critical, and progressing with related policies and activities therefore became less important. Further, as evidenced by the publications and reports produced throughout this period, it is clear that even though the WHO secretariat identified influenza as a 'major threat' in its 2001 report to the 54th WHA on global health security (WHO 2001d), equally the secretariat continued to largely view the disease as a public health problem that could be addressed by conventional public health measures – influenza-as-a-security-threat had still not been widely internalized. Added to this, the appointment of a new director-general in 1998 resulted in the organization undergoing a radical restructuring of its programmes and policies, which in turn unsettled some of its employees. Meanwhile, events outside the WHO – such as the 1997 Asian financial crisis, the launch of the MDGs, the 2001 terrorist attacks on the World Trade Centre and the Pentagon, and the Second Gulf War arguably also served to distract attention from the 'threat' of pandemic influenza, reducing the perceived urgency to deal with the issue amongst both the organization's principals and the agent itself. Although it would be unfair to label such an outcome as IO shirking, it is equally the case that the WHO secretariat was afforded more time and space to pursue its influenza-related delegated responsibilities – time and space that the agent willingly took advantage of, that is, until events again overtook the IO.

Confirmation in early 2004 of widespread outbreaks of H5N1 avian influenza throughout several East Asian countries fundamentally changed the WHO's approach to influenza. Moreover, since 2004 the organization's global influenza programme has remained in a state of perpetual alert. This is principally because, as the WHO secretariat has noted, H5N1 and the more recent H7N9 avian influenza virus that emerged in March 2013 retain 'pandemic potential, because they continue to circulate widely in some poultry populations, most humans likely have no immunity to them, and they can cause severe disease and death in humans' (WHO 2014e). Although at the time of writing neither the H5N1 virus nor the H7N9 virus has successfully transmuted into a pathogen that spreads easily between humans, the potential hazard nevertheless remains, and the WHO secretariat continues to closely monitor the situation.

Intriguingly, the first reappearance of the H5N1 influenza virus after the 1997 outbreak in Hong Kong coincided with the emergence of the 2003 SARS outbreak. In February 2003 two human cases were confirmed, and a third was later suspected, resulting in two fatalities (WHO 2011b). The virus temporarily disappeared again for a number of months, until November that year, when it again re-emerged in China to cause the death of yet another individual. Over the next few months further human infections continued to occur sporadically, but as early as February 2004 the virus was confirmed to be infecting poultry in over nine territories throughout East and Southeast Asia (ibid.), indicating that the virus had gained a firm epidemiological foothold throughout the region. By mid-2005 the virus had expanded its purchase, progressively spreading to Central Asia, Europe, Africa, and the Middle East (WHO 2006b).

Bolstered from its successful management of the 2003 SARS outbreak, the WHO secretariat responded forcefully to the new menace. Since February 2003, both the GISN and the GOARN had been attuned to the potential reappearance of the H5N1 virus, and when this was then confirmed in November that same year, both networks went on full alert. Through the GISN the secretariat was kept apprised of the changing epidemiological situation in Asia as official notifications and data were received from NICs, national ministries of health, and WHO epidemiologists in the field (WHO 2006b). This data in turn permitted the organization to again start providing policy advice in real-time, which it accomplished via the GOARN's disease outbreak news website and the *Weekly Epidemiological Record*. It is in this regard that the WHO secretariat also revisited its role as a directing and coordinating authority, for as soon as the epidemiological picture indicated that the virus had gained a foothold in Asia the organization responded by urging member states to develop pandemic preparedness plans, increase surveillance, and strengthen their health systems to be more responsive. Unlike the WHO's management of SARS, however, the organization somewhat ameliorated its approach. For whilst the WHO directed member states to take actions designed 'to strengthen national preparedness, reduce opportunities for a pandemic virus to emerge, improve the early warning system, delay initial international spread and accelerate vaccine development', and closely monitored their progress in following this advice (WHO 2005b, p. 384), the secretariat did not criticize or condemn those countries that failed to do so.

The WHO secretariat's approach and response to the reappearance of the H5N1 virus – at least in its initial days – thus exemplified a combination of the organization's classical approach to disease eradication and its newfound, emboldened method. For instance, the WHO secretariat assumed the function of real-time epidemic intelligence coordinator, gathering data from its principals affected by the virus, identifying gaps in existing knowledge and evidence, and promoting further research be undertaken. Similarly, it performed an effective role in acting as a real-time policy adviser, issuing recommendations and advice on what governments could do to mitigate the H5N1 threat. It is in this regard that the WHO secretariat also employed a more confident tone in its communications with its principals, returning to its constitutionally mandated role as the directing and coordinating authority by instructing member states to implement a series of measures as rapidly as possible. Where the organization deviated substantially, however, from its post-SARS approach was in again declining to serve as government assessor and critic.

What explains this break with the WHO's newly minted approach to managing global health security? Conceivably there may be a number of explanations. Arguably the first is that the reappearance of the H5N1 virus coincided with a series of regional consultations on the revised IHR (ahead of the formal IGWG) whereby the WHO's powers and authority were again under review. Although member states had unanimously publicly praised the organization's handling of the SARS outbreak at the 56th WHA in May 2003, privately concerns were being raised in the lead up to the IHR IGWG about the level and extent of IO autonomy that the WHO secretariat had displayed. Several countries, including Canada, Norway, Russia, Switzerland, Samoa, and the United States responded to early drafts of the proposed legislative framework, highlighting the need to carefully balance the WHO's imperative to intervene in a public health emergency with state sovereignty, with many erring on the side of protecting principals' sovereignty. The fact that so many member states expressed reservations – even those who were widely viewed as 'WHO friendly', such as Norway – regarding the level of the IO's autonomy undoubtedly sent a clear message to the secretariat that it needed to proceed with caution or risk a backlash from its principals through the imposition of new control mechanisms.

A second potential explanation for why the WHO secretariat refrained from publicly criticizing member states may be simply that so few of them had taken steps to protect themselves. By the organization's own reckoning, for instance, by 2005 less than 25 per cent of member states had even developed pandemic preparedness plans despite six years of the IO's urging, and even fewer had actually taken steps to gain access to anti-viral drugs (WHO 2005b, p. 384). For the WHO secretariat to roundly criticize three quarters of its member states would hardly have served much benefit. Any perceived criticisms would likely have antagonized the organization's distal and proximal principals alike and again risked the possibility that member states would retaliate, either by reducing the IO's operational budget or by applying new legal constraints.

The third possibility that may have affected the WHO secretariat's willingness to criticize member states at this time was the proposed creation of an entirely new entity: the United Nations System Influenza Coordinator (UNSIC). By early 2005 multiple UN and non-UN agencies – such as the Food and Agriculture Organization (FAO), the UNDP, UNICEF, the World Bank, and the World Organization for Animal Health (OIE), amongst others – had launched programmes targeting H5N1. Concerns were subsequently expressed within the UN (and later by several Asian leaders) that some of these programmes might work at cross-purposes and place unduly heavy reporting burdens on recipient countries. In addition, it was recognized that the UN itself lacked a contingency plan for responding to a pandemic, and so a meeting was convened in New York on 13 September 2005, involving several senior UN officials and associated agencies engaged in H5N1 work, to discuss the creation of a coordinating entity.

For the WHO secretariat the establishment of another purpose-built UN agency to deal with a specific disease likely caused anxiety that its authority in global health would again be compromised. As noted earlier, the perceived failure of the IO's leadership in responding to the emergence of HIV/AIDS was widely attributed to the creation of UNAIDS in 1996, which assumed the WHO's mandate for coordinating global efforts to combat the disease. In 2005 when the proposal was then put forward to create an entirely new entity for responding to the menace of pandemic influenza, WHO Director-General Dr Jong-wook Lee met with UN Secretary General Kofi Annan to discuss the terms of UNSIC's role and responsibilities, no doubt in part to prevent a repeat of history and the possibility that the WHO would be circumvented. David Nabarro, who was appointed to lead UNSIC in September 2005 (UN 2014a), recalls:

> Obviously staff in WHO wondered what my role and theirs would be because it was a new position. But the terms of reference for my job were very much jointly decided by Kofi Annan and Jong-wook Lee to firstly help the UN system prepare for a pandemic, and secondly to help UN agencies as a whole work in support of countries on pandemic preparedness but always with the technical direction being provided by WHO. UNSIC was also always a tiny outfit, and I was just one person, so I was absolutely clear that our job was just to coordinate and to take the technical guidance of WHO and promote it amongst all relevant UN agencies including those tasked with development, humanitarian and peacekeeping responsibilities. (Nabarro 2014)

Lastly, a number of factors within the organization may also explain – at least to some degree – why the WHO secretariat declined to serve as government assessor and critic in the case of H5N1. For instance, in July 2003 the new WHO director-general, Dr Jong-wook Lee, removed Dr David Heymann from his role as executive director of the Communicable Diseases Cluster (the unit which had coordinated the WHO's response to SARS) and appointed him as Special Representative to the Director-General for Polio Eradication. This transfer was widely interpreted by staff within the WHO as an admonishment to Dr Heymann and an attempt by the director-general to appease disgruntled member states (Anonymous 2005).[1] Arguably, however, Dr Lee's actions also reflected a different management style from that of the former director-general, Dr Gro Harlem Brundtland, who was perceived as 'a calculated risk taker' (Heymann 2005). Ultimately though, irrespective of which set of circumstances best explains why the WHO secretariat refrained from assessing and/or criticizing member states, it is clear that in the context of H5N1 the IO altered its management approach again, returning to its pre-SARS respectful deference towards member states.

Moreover, this revised approach permeated the WHO's efforts towards H5N1 even as the organization intensified its securitization of the disease. In November 2005, for example, the WHO hosted a joint intergovernmental meeting (IGM) on H5N1 with the World Bank, the OIE, and the FAO. The meeting, which brought together over 600 experts from more than 100 countries, sought to take stock of efforts to date in combating the virus and to heighten awareness of the need for decisive measures and additional resources (WHO 2005c). To accomplish the latter, the threat of another influenza pandemic was repeatedly emphasized, with many participants reportedly noting that 'pandemic influenza was a threat with scientific, technical, political, social, economic, agricultural, and health dimensions as well as implications for national and global security' (ibid., p. 9). While various governments, international agencies, and NGOs were acknowledged as having a role to play in H5N1 containment efforts, the WHO – or more specifically, its real-time epidemic intelligence coordinator role – was viewed as critical. As the summary report noted, 'Clear information about the evolving epidemiological situation was also essential to allow WHO to declare the right level of pandemic alert, which, in turn, would trigger a defined series of national and international response measures' (ibid., p. 24). Likewise, despite the fact that the UNSIC office was now officially responsible for global coordination, in reality the WHO secretariat lost little of its directing and coordinating authority via issuing real-time policy advice. Unlike SARS, however, the WHO secretariat did not publicly comment on or criticize member states that failed to follow its guidelines. Rather, the IO preferred to emphasize the need for further action against the H5N1 'threat' and sought constructive collaboration with H5N1-affected countries at the regional, national, and sub-national levels (WHO 2005d, Curley and Herington 2011, Phommasack et al. 2012).

One of the key recommendations to emerge from the November 2005 meeting was for member states to voluntarily comply with the revised IHR (2005). Even though the framework had only been endorsed less than six months previously, in light of the spread of H5N1 participants at the meeting voiced their strong support in urging member states to act as if the revised IHR already applied (WHO 2005c, pp. 27, 30). The WHO secretariat, acting on this recommendation, subsequently invited all member states to establish liaison offices (otherwise described as 'National Focal Points' [NFPs] under the revised IHR) and initiated a process to establish an Influenza Pandemic Task Force (akin to the IHR Emergency Committee provision under the IHR [2005]) to provide strategic advice. These measures were then formally endorsed in May the following year with the passage of resolution *WHA59.2 Application of the International Health Regulations (2005)*. The resolution also directed the secretariat to mobilize international assistance and financial resources in aiding member states to build and strengthen their health systems, develop guidelines, stockpile pharmaceuticals, and accelerate training in surveillance, biosafety, and laboratory capacity (WHO 2006c, pp. 3–6). The pandemic task force then met for the first time in September 2006 to provide expert advice on avian and pandemic influenza and to recommend the WHO pandemic alert level (WHO 2006d).

The November IGM reflected the fact that, by 2005, the international community had become particularly alarmed by the spread of the H5N1 virus and its potential to instigate an influenza pandemic – an unease that ultimately only dissipated with the commencement of the 2009 H1N1 influenza pandemic. Throughout this period, the WHO secretariat proved central in aiding its principals to respond to the perceived crisis, gathering surveillance data and publishing results, issuing new pandemic influenza preparedness guidelines (WHO 2005e), extending and improving geographical information systems for disease surveillance (WHO 2006d), launching operational protocols for rapid response, developing strategic action plans, lobbying for additional financial resources, developing stockpiles of drugs and an action plan for increasing vaccine supply, and offering training courses (WHO 2007e). The secretariat also played a prominent role internationally, working closely with other IOs such as the FAO, the OIE, the World Bank, and UNSIC to ensure coordination and avoid duplication of effort (see, for example, FAO and OIE 2007, IMCAPI 2008), as well as regionally with organizations such as the Association of South East Asian Nations (ASEAN) and the European Commission to help strengthen preparedness (EC 2010). The organization thus executed its mandate as the coordinating authority in international health matters, as well as its real-time epidemic intelligence coordinator and policy adviser roles, but continued to shirk its directing authority and eschew any perceived or actual criticism of member states' performance.

Alongside the WHO secretariat's technical assistance, the organization was also engaged in an active campaign to reframe influenza not just as a public health menace, but also as a threat to national and international security. This threat narrative surrounding influenza had begun a decade earlier, but by 2005 the WHO secretariat had fully embraced this new rhetoric (Davies 2008, Kamradt-Scott and McInnes 2012, Weir 2015). Moreover, as reflected in the WHO's 2005 pandemic preparedness guidelines, the organization clearly viewed the securitization of the disease as a strategic tool, noting, 'A new appreciation of infectious diseases as threats to global and national security offers the prospect that high-level political leadership could be enlisted in support of the necessary intersectoral planning' (WHO 2005e, p. 4). Some members of the WHO secretariat have been even more explicit, as Andrew Cassels, former Director of Strategy for the Office of the Director-General, noted in an interview in 2010, stating:

> The security and economic arguments have gone hand in hand. First of all it was about bringing HIV/AIDS to the forefront of the agenda, but then it expanded to include deliberate release. In part though, it has also been about securing political and financial support for the organisation. Bringing health issues into the security domain has been a fairly deliberate strategy – one that has been criticized by some Member States admittedly, but one that has probably been inevitable. (Interview on 22 March 2010, as quoted in Kamradt-Scott and McInnes 2012, p. S101)

Subsequent reports produced by the WHO secretariat for member states' consumption – either in the WHA or the EB meetings – habitually emphasized not only the physical dangers, but also the economic, social, and political threats the disease presented (WHO EB 2006a, WHO 2007e, 2008c). In November 2006 the newly appointed director-general, Dr Margaret Chan, identified the 'looming threat of an influenza pandemic' as a particular menace to global health security (WHO EB 2006a, p. 3), but the following year the securitization of the disease was escalated even further with the publication of the 2007 World Health Report that identified pandemic influenza as 'the most feared security threat' (WHO 2007a, p. 45). The intended audience of the WHO's securitization attempts – namely its member states – responded in kind, with the majority of countries developing pandemic preparedness plans, implementing 'all hazards' and 'one health' contingency planning, stockpiling pharmacological products, and changing legislation to facilitate prompt reporting (see, for example, Elbe 2011, Martin and Conseil 2012, Mwacalimba and Green 2014). In a few instances, governments even responded by ranking pandemic influenza as a more serious threat to national security than terrorism (Elbe et al. 2014). Although the WHO secretariat was not the only IO to engage in securitizing moves by repeatedly describing and emphasizing the 'threat' influenza posed (see IMF 2006, UNSIC 2006, FAO and OIE 2007), equally, due to its prominence in the global response to H5N1 and its recognized authority on international health matters, the IO was indubitably at the forefront of securitizing actors, advocating not only for new emergency powers (in the form of the revised IHR), but also for additional resources to combat the threat.

The 2009 H1N1 influenza pandemic

Surprisingly, however, the first influenza pandemic of the 21st century did not arise from the much-feared H5N1 virus, but instead emerged from an influenza strain usually found in pigs. Even more unexpectedly, the pandemic spread globally from a small Mexican village in La Gloria, Veracruz, as opposed from somewhere within Asia, which for many years has been viewed as a 'hot bed' of emerging infectious diseases and where the bulk of H5N1 human cases had occurred. Exactly when the influenza A(H1N1) strain achieved human-to-human transmission is not entirely known (Girard et al. 2010), but the virus was detected in early March 2009 when the Mexican Ministry of Health received reports of an unusually high number of individuals experiencing influenza-like illness when seasonal influenza cases were expected to be in decline. Unsure of whether the cases were an anomaly or something more serious, the Mexican Directorate General of Epidemiology ordered that surveillance for acute respiratory diseases be heightened. Throughout the first 10 days of April 2009, government and non-government sources then began to document an outbreak of an influenza-like illness that had affected a large proportion of La Gloria's inhabitants (Brown 2009, WHO 2009a, Shkabatur 2011). Samples collected from patients identified an influenza A virus but the sub-type was unknown, and so under a newly agreed health security pact between the United States, Mexico, and Canada, the specimens were sent to the CDC in Atlanta and the Canadian Public Health Agency's National Microbiology Laboratory for testing. On 18 April the CDC notified the WHO under the IHR (2005) to the presence of a novel strain of influenza with human-to-human transmission (PAHO 2009a, WHO 2009a), but the virus had already spread to Mexico City, the United States, and Canada (WHO 2009a, Davies et al. 2015).

The international community responded vigorously and rapidly to this news. Somewhat ironically, even as the virus was infecting villagers in Mexico, in Geneva the WHO secretariat was planning a simulation exercise to test the IHR (2005) framework. Confronted with the presence of a new influenza strain with pandemic potential the exercise was understandably abandoned as real-life events overtook the IO and international attention fixated on the evolving epidemiological situation in Mexico. In contrast to China's actions during the SARS outbreak, the Mexican government openly shared information regarding the number of cases and the measures they were taking to limit the pathogen's spread. As a result, by late April 2009 Mexican health authorities had conveyed to the WHO – and the wider international community – that infection rates had reached as high as 50 per cent in some areas (WHO 2009b), that there were over 1,300 suspected cases, and that 84 deaths could probably be attributed to the new influenza strain (PAHO 2009b). Several countries, including China, Argentina, Peru, Cuba, Sudan, and Ecuador reacted negatively to this information by imposing temporary bans on all flights from Mexico, while others resorted to quarantining Mexican and/or other North American citizens (Gostin 2009, Hodge 2010, Katz and Fischer 2010). When further information came to light that the virus was of porcine origin, prompting the WHO secretariat to initially label the disease 'Swine Flu', over 20 countries responded by imposing trade import bans on pork and pork products while other countries such as Egypt and Iraq resorted to slaughtering livestock (Karadesh 2009, Katz and Fischer 2010).

Nonetheless, the virus continued to spread. Invoking the IHR (2005) framework for the first time, WHO Director-General Margaret Chan officially convened the inaugural meeting of the IHR Emergency Committee on 25 April 2009 to provide guidance on the rapidly changing epidemiological situation. On the basis of the Committee's first assessment, the WHO's pandemic alert phase was increased from level 3 (limited human-to-human transmission) to level 4 (community-level outbreaks) on 27 April 2009. Just two days later it was raised again, this time to level 5 (sustained community transmission) following laboratory confirmation of localized outbreaks occurring within nine countries (WHO 2009c). Over the next fortnight, the WHO secretariat executed its now well-trodden real-time epidemic intelligence coordinator and policy adviser roles by gathering data and reports, holding regular press briefings, and issuing daily – at times twice daily – global updates and alerts containing medical guidance and recommendations. Moreover, in this capacity, by 12 May the secretariat had obtained official reports of some 5,251 confirmed cases of influenza A(H1N1) throughout 30 countries in the Americas, Europe, and Oceania (WHO 2009a).

Despite these figures, by early May 2009 the WHO secretariat was criticized for having acted prematurely in declaring pandemic alert phase 5. According to the WHO's latest pandemic guidelines that had been released only a few months earlier, the declaration of phase 5 was meant to be 'a strong signal that a pandemic is imminent' (WHO 2009d, p. 25), which was also expected to cause severe illness and large numbers of human deaths. The epidemiological picture that was emerging, however, suggested that the H1N1 virus did not meet these criteria; yet when the IO was questioned over this apparent disjuncture between its guidelines and the seemingly mild nature of the virus, the secretariat responded by removing its latest guidelines from its website (Cohen 2009). Not surprisingly, these actions created disquiet amongst the IO's principals, so much so that the WHO director-general convened an urgent high-level consultation immediately prior to the scheduled 2009 WHA to examine the IHR Emergency Committee's decisions and the available epidemiological data, with the aim of reassuring member states that its response to H1N1 was both measured and appropriate (WHO 2009e). Nonetheless, throughout the WHA the political pressure applied by the IO's principals became so intense that Dr Keiji Fukuda, director of the WHO Influenza Programme, subsequently announced that the organization would include a new severity assessment in its definition of a pandemic (McNeil 2009, SooHoo 2009, Doshi 2011).

In response to member states' calls for greater transparency and clarity, the WHO director-general convened the IHR Emergency Committee for a third time on 5 June to obtain advice on whether to amend the IO's definition of a pandemic and whether the continued spread of the virus now warranted declaration of a full-scale pandemic (phase 6). Some 64 countries had already reported at least one laboratory-confirmed case of H1N1 (WHO 2009f); yet while the Committee determined that further announcements ought to discuss severity issues wherever possible, it advised against raising the current pandemic alert status (WHO 2009d). The following week, however, this decision was overturned when, confronted by over 28,100 laboratory-confirmed cases, 144 H1N1-related deaths, and sustained community-level outbreaks throughout multiple countries, the Committee recommended the director-general raise the global alert status to reflect the fact that a full-scale pandemic was underway (Davies et al. 2015). Dutifully following this advice, Dr Chan announced the first influenza pandemic of the 21st century on 11 June 2009 (WHO 2009g).

Over the ensuing weeks and months the WHO secretariat performed its dual role as real-time epidemic intelligence coordinator and policy adviser with exactitude, providing regular updates on the ever-changing epidemiological situation and outlining in considerable detail the severity of the pandemic throughout different areas, countries, and regions. Indeed, it was on the basis of the IO's constant accumulation and interpretation of epidemiological data that the director-general was subsequently empowered to declare, on 10 August 2010, that the international community had now entered the 'post-pandemic period' (WHO 2010a), officially signalling the end to the H1N1 pandemic. Throughout this period the organization had also continued to issue medical advice and recommendations on how best to treat suspected or confirmed cases (WHO 2009h, 2009i), the inappropriateness of trade and travel restrictions (WHO 2009j), and the availability and usefulness of pharmaceutical countermeasures (WHO 2009k, 2009l). Interim guideline documents were likewise produced on surveillance protocols (WHO 2009m), communication strategies (WHO 2009n), and social distancing measures such as school closures (WHO 2009o).

It was additionally in this regard that the WHO was clearly viewed by its member states as the lead technical agency in coordinating the international community's efforts to combat the spread of the H1N1 virus. Yet once again the IO sought to avoid the perception that it was directing its principals. Throughout the organization's communications and policy advice to member states, for instance, the WHO secretariat abjured an overly prescriptive approach, selecting instead to outline a series of actions, principles, and preferred measures that member states *should* apply – if they chose to do so – to counter the spread of the virus within their respective territories (see, for example, WHO 2009p, 2009q). Within this context, the organization did not shy from indicating the limits of acceptable state behaviour; but equally, in seeking to provide member states with options that took account of the available scientific evidence and their respective economic, social, and epidemiological circumstances, the IO also sought to avoid the risk that its leadership might be viewed as inflexible.

At the broader global level the organization also assumed a lead role in coordinating other public and private entities engaged in H1N1-related work. Although officially UNSIC was tasked with coordinating all UN agencies' efforts, in reality the office of the Coordinator lacked the human resource capacity to mount a far-reaching campaign and so, by necessity, focused its energies on addressing urgent needs via the implementation of a system to aid low-income countries (Nabarro 2014). Aware of UNSIC's limitations, the WHO secretariat unashamedly took responsibility for coordinating the various UN agencies such as the OIE and the FAO (WHO 2009r), yet was equally conscious to at least publicly declare in a joint statement with the International Federation of the Red Cross, UNSIC, OCHA, and UNICEF that 'No one agency can provide all of priority interventions. Instead they should be coordinated by building on capacities and comparative advantages of each partner' (WHO 2009s). Using the vehicle of a speech to the UN General Assembly at the commencement of the pandemic, the WHO director-general also sought to apply political pressure to pharmaceutical manufacturers to donate a proportion of their products to low-income countries (WHO 2009t). In the months that followed, multiple private meetings and consultation discussions were held, which proved partially successful (see WHO 2009u). Throughout these various interventions, however, the WHO secretariat was careful to avoid the risk of alienating organizations and entities by seeming overly prescriptive or aggressive, preferring instead to coordinate efforts where there was consensus and emphasize the need for all parties to work together towards a common purpose.

Even so, the WHO's handling of the crisis did attract further criticism. In late 2009, a Danish newspaper alleged that members of the IHR Emergency Committee had received financial support from pharmaceutical manufacturers. The charge, which implied that the director-general had been improperly influenced into declaring a PHEIC, provoked the secretariat to publicly release the names of the scientists and public health experts serving on the Committee. It also occasioned the director-general to issue a strongly worded statement refuting the allegations, reaffirming, 'The world is going through a real pandemic. The description of it as a fake is wrong and irresponsible' (WHO 2010b). The statement nonetheless proved insufficient to dispel public disquiet, and both the Council of Europe and the *British Medical Journal* initiated inquiries to ascertain whether the WHO had been improperly influenced into declaring a pandemic. In April 2010, before the findings of these inquiries were handed down, the director-general announced that an additional, independent external review would be held to examine the WHO's management of the 2009 H1N1 pandemic and appointed Dr Harvey Fineberg from the US Institute of Medicine to oversee the investigation (Davìes et al. 2015). Although the inquiries ultimately failed to identify any improper conduct, Director-General Chan accepted the need to review the organization's policies and procedures in light of the criticisms that emerged (WHO 2011c), resulting in several reports to the WHA detailing the measures taken (WHO 2012a, 2012b, 2013a, 2014f).

It could be appreciated, therefore, that unlike the 2003 SARS outbreak the 2009 H1N1 pandemic was not a resounding political success for the WHO secretariat in spite of its epidemiological outcome. The IO's handling of the crisis was heavily criticized from several directions over a perceived lack of openness and transparency in the secretariat's decision-making processes. These criticisms adversely affected the WHO secretariat's credibility, evidenced by the fact that no less than three external investigations were launched to establish whether corporate interests had unduly influenced the IO. The criticisms levelled at the WHO secretariat also had two further consequences, serving to firstly divert the secretariat's attention and energy into defending the organization and, secondly, to make the IO even less willing to criticize a select number of member states that openly – and in some instances, unapologetically – contravened the IHR (2005) agreement.

As noted earlier, for example, following the revelation that a novel influenza virus with pandemic potential of Mexican origin was spreading internationally, a number of countries responded by quarantining Mexican citizens and travellers from Mexico, irrespective of whether or not they were exhibiting any symptoms of the disease. Some other governments cancelled all international flights to and from Mexico, with a few even extending equivalent bans to all flights from North America. Added to this, in the wake of the WHO secretariat's decision to label the disease 'swine flu' on 24 April 2009 (presumably to avoid the risk that it would become known as the 'Mexican Flu' and the damage that would ensue to Mexico's economy were that association to affix), several governments immediately applied importation bans on live pigs and pork products, and a small number slaughtered existing livestock. As soon as this information came to light, the WHO secretariat attempted to counter these measures by issuing a statement on 27 April 2009 that travel restrictions were not warranted and that there was no risk of infection 'from consumption of well-cooked pork and pork products' (WHO 2009j). Yet despite that these statements were reissued and intermittently repeated (WHO 2009v), and although the WHO secretariat refrained from ever again referring to the disease as 'swine flu' from 29 April onwards, throughout the pandemic approximately 20 to 30 countries retained these trade import bans on pork and pork products.

Not surprisingly, countries that were large pork exporters immediately decried the bans, citing the need to ensure measures were based on scientific evidence as stipulated in the revised IHR – evidence, critically, which was absent. Yet while other member states joined with the pork-exporting countries in condemning the actions of those that imposed the bans (Davies et al. 2015), rather than join with the majority of its principals the WHO secretariat elected instead to simply reiterate its earlier statements on the safety of well-cooked pork and pork products. This, it has to be said, was to many a somewhat unexpected development, given the forcefulness with which the WHO secretariat had responded to China's actions throughout SARS and given the fact that under the IHR (2005) the IO had been officially imbued – for the first time – with the authority to publicly 'name and shame' countries that did not comply with the object and purpose of the revised cooperation framework. Equally, however, when viewed against the IO's traditional reluctance to criticize or even be perceived to be critical of its member states, the WHO secretariat's actions were entirely consistent with the organization's classical approach to disease eradication. The corollary of the secretariat's reticence to utilize its new 'name and shame' powers, left those countries adversely affected by the trade and travel bans little recourse other than to raise their objections within the context of the WTO's dispute resolution forum (WTO 2011).

So what explains the WHO secretariat's feeble defence of the revised IHR (2005) framework and its unwillingness to defend its newly fortified global health security authority? Conceivably, as in the case of the WHO's management of the H5N1 crisis, a variety of internal and external factors may have been involved. For example, a large proportion of the countries that applied trade importation bans on pork and pork products were observed to comprise Muslim-majority populations. Although it remains unlikely to have been the only cause, it nevertheless may have been that the WHO secretariat refrained from publicly criticizing member states, fearing that any criticisms might be interpreted as anti-Islamic and/or religiously motivated. For an IO that is fiercely protective of its assumed impartial, apolitical reputation, such an outcome would be especially damaging and therefore worth avoiding.

Another important consideration may have been the identity of those member states that applied excessive additional health measures and their pre-existing relationship with the WHO. One of the countries, for instance, that instituted trade import bans (as well as taking the rather unusual measure of slaughtering its entire pig population following the announcement that the virus was of porcine origin) was Egypt. Yet, since the 1950s, Egypt has hosted the WHO regional office for the Eastern Mediterranean (EMRO) and in this role has often sought to serve as a regional leader in advocating compliance with the IO's programmes, policies, and procedures. In this regard, for many years Egypt has operated as a proximal principal to the WHO secretariat, and the IO may have been justifiably concerned that its severe criticism of those member states that contravened the IHR (2005) protocols might further antagonize the Egyptian government and thereby damage relations with EMRO.

Similarly, another country that was observed to apply trade import bans on pork and pork products was Indonesia, which since 2007 had enjoyed a somewhat strained relationship with the WHO secretariat over what was described as 'a breakdown of mutual trust' (Sedyaningsih et al. 2008). The dispute between Indonesia and the WHO paradoxically arose as a direct consequence of the securitization of pandemic influenza and was eventually resolved (see Elbe 2010a, Kamradt-Scott 2013), but in 2009, at the height of the H1N1 influenza pandemic, tensions remained. Indonesia, like Egypt, had also actively cultivated its regional leadership credentials, including (as will be explored in greater depth in the next chapter) adopting an adversarial position towards the WHO's reframing of its public health mandate under a security rubric. Accordingly, the WHO secretariat may have been concerned that strident criticisms of any government's actions may further harm not only its direct relationship with Indonesia, but also the IO's engagement with other countries in the region.

A third possible explanation may be that the WHO secretariat, aware of the lack of enforcement mechanisms to ensure member state compliance with the IHR (2005), simply decided that it was powerless to affect any change in behaviour. Admittedly, this account is probably considered the least plausible, if only for the fact that the WHO secretariat had worked so tirelessly to see the IHR – and by implication, its own global health security authority and powers – revised and updated. It would also be inconsistent with the decade-long trajectory of the WHO secretariat actively seeking to influence state behaviour via the promotion, adoption, and internalization of new global health security norms (see Davies et al. 2015). Having said this, it must be acknowledged that by 2009 several members of the WHO secretariat's epistemic community that had been so instrumental in promoting the IO's new risk management approach – individuals such as David Heymann, Mike Ryan, Sandy Cocksedge, Guénaël Rodier, and others – had either left the IO entirely or moved portfolios, resulting in a change of personnel that may have held different views on the ability of the WHO to affect change.

Arguably, the most compelling explanation is that the WHO secretariat had internalized the lessons learned from SARS and adopted a 'small target' approach to prevent further principal retaliation. The director-general must have been aware, for instance, of the extent to which even 'friendly' member states had expressed concern over the level of IO autonomy displayed by the WHO in the context of SARS and the measures then taken collectively by principals throughout the IHR IGWG to prevent a repeat of such behaviour. More specifically, although at the time the majority of member states were supportive of the WHO secretariat's public critique of the Chinese government over its attempted subterfuge and mishandling of SARS, equally no member state wanted to be subjected to a similar experience. This led directly to the new requirement under the IHR (2005) for the director-general to convene an IHR Emergency Committee comprised of government-nominated experts with which s/he is obliged to consult. Against this background, it is entirely plausible that the WHO secretariat was reluctant to risk antagonizing even a small proportion of member states in the context of the 2009 H1N1 pandemic – irrespective of whether they were proximal or distal principals – over fear that it might lead to retribution and a further reduction of IO autonomy and authority. In such a scenario, the director-general may very well have weighed the costs and benefits involved and determined that strident criticism of governments over their adoption of excessive (albeit limited) additional health measures was simply not in the long-term interests of the WHO.

Of course, even if the above account is considered the most credible, it is nevertheless conjectural. What is important to appreciate is that the WHO secretariat's actions – or more specifically, lack of action – in condemning those member states that flagrantly contravened the IHR (2005) during the H1N1 pandemic fundamentally undermined the revised framework at its very first investiture. If, as suppositioned above, the director-general did favour protecting the IO's post-IGWG autonomy over and above the revised IHR, then regrettably it was done so at the cost of the very framework the WHO secretariat had worked so hard to re-establish.

Conclusion

As this chapter has sought to highlight, the WHO secretariat's first attempts to respond to the menace of pandemic influenza very much reflected the IO's classical approach to disease eradication. Indeed, when the WHO secretariat established the governance structures in the 1950s to monitor the disease, they were designed explicitly in such a way as to help the IO consolidate the available epidemiological intelligence, which it would then disseminate via weekly publication. While the organization's policy advice to governments was initially very limited due to the uncertain benefit of influenza vaccines, intriguingly, when the efficacy of pharmacological interventions was proven, the WHO secretariat immediately sought to divest (shirk) some of its responsibilities for global management of the threat by encouraging member states to build pharmaceutical manufacturing capacity and thereby take ownership of the problem. Critically, however, during most of the 20th century the WHO secretariat avoided evaluating member states' compliance with this advice. In this regard, the IO settled comfortably into its coordinating role, shunning the opportunity to direct, assess, or critique its principals on their performance.

By the late 1990s, however, a very different situation was emerging, which required the WHO to adjust its approach. The 1997 outbreak of

H5N1 in Hong Kong and its reappearance in the wake of SARS fed directly into a broader, now-established narrative of the 'threat' from emerging and re-emerging infectious diseases. In response, the WHO secretariat recognized that it needed to rapidly upscale its real-time epidemic intelligence, policy adviser, and overall coordination efforts. Moreover, as the chapter has evidenced, the WHO secretariat became acutely aware that this 'threat' narrative assisted in securing additional political attention and resources, and so, after initially testing the waters with the passage of resolution WHA54.14, the IO actively began to promulgate the securitization of public health hazards and particularly pandemic influenza. Member states, persuaded by the WHO secretariat's securitizing moves, allocated literally billions of dollars, passed new legislation, and amended existing or built new national, regional, and international governance structures to strengthen global pandemic preparedness. Within this context, the WHO was expected (and willingly assumed) a global coordination role despite the proliferation of actors now engaged in preparedness activities. Importantly, however, the IO was careful to avoid repeating its SARS-inspired role of government assessor and critic, as the reappearance of the pandemic influenza threat coincided with the IHR revision process in which the IO's autonomy and its new approach to managing global health security was being intensely scrutinized.

What the chapter has additionally sought to elicit is that in the wake of the IHR revision process the WHO's global health security mandate and its disease eradication delegation contract has once again undergone revision. On the one hand, the IO's principals intentionally used the IHR IGWG to impose a range of new control mechanisms on the WHO secretariat to prevent unintended IO autonomy and slippage. On the other hand, however, as evidenced by its actions in the context of the 2009 H1N1 influenza pandemic, the WHO secretariat – including, importantly, the director-general – appear to have constrained their own behaviour, presumably in an attempt to avoid the imposition of yet further limits on the organization's autonomy and/or amendments to its delegation contract. How these developments will manifest in the WHO secretariat's management of future public health emergencies remains decidedly unclear. But what is apparent is that while the WHO's adoption of the health security agenda was initially welcomed, in the wake of the IHR revision process there has been growing dissatisfaction amongst some principals over the secretariat's reframing exercise, which is the topic of the next chapter.

6
Global Health Security and Its Discontents

Since the initial deliberations in 1946 regarding the need for a new universal health organization, a strong correlation has existed between public health and international security. Having said this, the WHO secretariat's explicit adoption of security-related concepts and language to reframe its public health mandate is a fairly recent phenomenon that only emerged from 2001 onwards. Moreover, the WHO did not lead the charge to securitize public health – this was accomplished by a host of other actors. Admittedly, one of the WHO's proximal principals – the United States – was a key player in advocating this new way of viewing acute, fast-moving health issues (Smith III 2014), but the WHO secretariat itself lagged well behind, in some quarters even initially staunchly resisting the push to reframe public health in security terms. It is in this regard that the events of the mid-1990s, both within and external to the WHO, marked a distinct turning point. The WHO secretariat's advancement of the phrase 'global health security' in its 2001 report to member states signalled its firm embrace of this new worldview, and for more than a decade the WHO has been on the path of re-casting its public health mandate in a security frame.

Importantly, however, not everyone has welcomed the WHO's reframing efforts. Critics have emerged from a variety of quarters, but most notably from two distinct groups: academe; and even more disconcerting for the WHO secretariat, from a small but vocal sub-set of its member states. This chapter will examine the criticisms of the WHO's securitizing moves that have emerged, the purported benefits and drawbacks of such measures, and how the WHO secretariat has in turn responded by effectively attempting to now downplay, even desecuritize, its health-as-security mandate. The chapter then concludes with a discussion on what this trend may mean for the future and, in particular, how securitization's discontents may adversely affect – and potentially again re-shape – the WHO's new approach to managing global health security.

Securitization's discontents

It took some years after the WHO secretariat produced its 2001 report entitled *Global health security – epidemic alert and response* in which it argued for endorsement of GOARN and finalization of the IHR revision process to 'maintain global public health security' (WHO 2001d, p. 2, see also Fidler 2005), but criticisms have since emerged of the IO's decision to securitize its public health activities. As noted above, these critiques have emanated from two key groups of actors that include members of the global academic community and a limited but notably vocal sub-section of the WHO's member states.

A host of public health and politics/IR scholars have progressively materialized to criticize the fusion of health and security, noting various problems and potential dangers associated with securitization. Somewhat ironically, the bulk of academic critique has emerged from scholars based predominantly within high-income countries, and particularly from within the United Kingdom and the United States – two countries that have served as proximal principals to the WHO secretariat in strongly supporting the health-as-security agenda (UK Government 2008, WHO EB 2009, 2010a, 2013). While admittedly this trend indubitably reflects the power imbalances inherent within the academic profession, which in turn is reflective of a broader north–south divide (see Canagarajah 1996, Murphy and Zhu 2012), it is equally important to note that few criticisms of the health-as-security agenda have yet surfaced from scholarly communities located within the 'global south'.

By and large the criticisms that have appeared have generally followed three key trajectories. The first line of critique arises from Foucauldian and post-structuralist scholars that claim the health-as-security discourse is largely reflective of Western, high-income countries' neo-colonial predisposition towards protecting themselves against 'the rest'. Accordingly, by virtue of this fact, commentators such as King (2002), Ingram (2005), Collier and Lakoff (2008), Lakoff (2010), Lowe (2010), Abraham (2011), Stephenson (2012), and Stevenson and Moran (2015) advocate that the securitization of public health issues exposes yet another configuration of dominant interests manipulating and controlling the less powerful, replicating a form of governmentality and authority over the body politic. Often implicit within these critiques – and at times, less so – is the contention that because securitization predicates Western, high-income countries' interests above others, it is morally or ethically bankrupt. Yet others writers, such as Elbe (2010a, 2010b) and Elbe et al. (2014) trace that the securitization of health has had an equal and converse impact on security actors, leading to a medicalization, and even pharmaceuticalization, of the security sector.

A second common denunciation that often appears in the literature points to the potential distorting effects of the securitization of public health issues. In this, critics such as Greenberg (2002), Cohen et al. (2004), McInnes and Lee (2006), Aldis (2008), Rushton (2011), Youde (2012), and DeLaet (2015), amongst others, have pointed to the fact that the securitization of acute, fast-moving health issues (i.e. infectious diseases and/or bioweapons) has resulted in a disproportionate emphasis being placed on their prevention and control to the detriment of other, more pressing health matters. Even within the context of infectious disease outbreak control, scholars have pointed to the fact that some diseases attract more resources than others creating, in effect, a hierarchy of disease 'threats', with those that possess the ability to also threaten high-income countries commanding the greatest attention, while those that affect only the populations of low-income countries receiving considerably less. The underlying premise of these critiques is therefore one of social justice, which is recurrently aligned with the above critique of powerful interests manipulating the agenda.

The third line of critique that has emerged, which is often conflated with one or both of the above issues, is the actors (and their concomitant attitudes and authority) that securitization attracts. More specifically, concern amongst health-as-security detractors has tended to focus on the involvement of security sector personnel (i.e. police, military, intelligence) and the potential erosion of health/medical authority. The format in which such concerns are raised may vary, but usually takes the form of anxiety being expressed over the potential erosion of public health/humanitarian principles and/or human rights in order to respond effectively to the perceived 'threat' (see, for example, the arguments highlighted by Elbe 2006, Feldbaum et al. 2006, Calain 2007, Aldis 2008, Selgelid and Enemark 2008, Enemark 2009, McInnes and Rushton 2010, Ingram 2011, Smith 2013b). Importantly, however, the underlying cause of these concerns is the risk that by including non-health experts, the authority of medical/health professionals (as self-appointed guardians of these humanitarian principles and rights) and their ability to directly shape the response to a health problem will in some way become compromised, resulting in inadvertent or unintended outcomes.

Having said this, not all the antagonism towards the comingling of health and security has arisen from the health/humanitarian community and its supporters. On the converse side, although often more circumspect, security sector personnel have also been critical over what has been described as the 'medicalization' of security (see Elbe 2010a, 2010b), noting that health concerns are not 'core business' for the sector (Bernard 2013, p. 158). While such criticisms are understandable to a degree, equally they ignore the long historical association between military and security interests and the spread of disease (see, for example, Saengdidtha and Rangsin 2005, Bresalier 2011, Watterson and Kamradt-Scott 2015). Nonetheless, when viewed collectively, it is apparent that there continues to be widespread disquiet about the blurring of health and security boundaries, either due to the potential for unintended consequences, the intensification of existing inequalities and power imbalances, or the infringement of existing authority and principles.

Perhaps most intriguing is that amongst the wide variety of protagonists decrying the securitization of health, very few have taken aim at the WHO. This, it has to be acknowledged, is somewhat peculiar given that the WHO secretariat has been one of the most prominent securitizing actors of health issues. Indeed, as Stephenson (2012, p. 97) observes, securitization has now become so dominant that 'security is not presented as a mere dimension of or justification for the work of public health; it *is* public health' (emphasis original). Yet while some commentators initially criticized the WHO secretariat for its management of the 2003 SARS outbreak, arguing that its actions constituted IO agency slack (Fidler 2004, Cortell and Peterson 2006), its actions in securitizing health issues has attracted very little direct criticism. Even those academics who have adopted a more critical perspective have been rather muted in their reproach of the WHO. For instance, Stevenson and Moran (2015, p. 331) have noted in their work that the advancement of the health-as-security agenda has placed the IO in an 'awkward position of shifting the basis for investing in disease surveillance programs from humanitarian grounds towards safeguarding national security and international trade'. Yet even though these authors go on to question whose interests are served by the WHO's narrow definition of health security (ibid., pp. 332–336), the organization itself escapes further rebuke. Oswald (2011, p. 28) has similarly observed that the WHO secretariat has 'promoted a narrow and state-centered health security concept that was also influenced by the events of 11th September 2001, and by the potential threats of biological weapons and terrorism'. Here again though, while Oswald goes on to advocate for a broadening and deepening of the

WHO's conceptualization of health security, additional direct criticism of the IO responsible is absent.

Likewise, in their work Jin and Karackattu (2011, p. 181) have noted that the WHO secretariat has benefitted considerably from the securitization of health in terms of additional powers and authority, but that 'it may be counterproductive to global health governance'. In more precise terms, noting the actions of specific members of the WHO secretariat (including former Director-General Brundtland) in securitizing infectious diseases, these scholars argue:

> By strengthening global surveillance, [the] WHO consolidates its authoritative role and normative power and developed countries win enough time to take preventive and pre-emptive measures against infectious diseases spreading from developing countries. The recognition that [the] WHO's surveillance prioritizes the security concerns of developed countries dampens the intention of developing countries to cooperate with [the] WHO, rendering problematic the efficacy of the surveillance system. (ibid., p. 185)

Jin and Karackattu (ibid.) further contend that the 'WHO's securitization of infectious diseases . . . is not motivated by global health promotion but by the narrow security interests of developed countries'. Beyond these comments, however, the WHO secretariat largely evades further blame for its securitization activities. Rather, the authors stress at multiple junctures that the secretariat 'has been trying to keep itself away from sensitive security issues' (ibid., p. 182, see also pp. 181, 184).

To date, the two notable exceptions to this trend have been the works of Davies (2008) and Hanrieder and Kreuder-Sonnen (2014). In her work, Davies (2008, p. 296) asserts that 'the WHO has been a primary actor in constructing the emerging discourse of infectious disease securitization, and western states in particular have been quick to engage with this discourse'. Davies goes on to argue that both the IO and developed states have directly benefited from the health-as-security frame, with high-income countries using the organization as a shield to help protect their own citizens, while the WHO has strengthened its credentials as the paramount authority in global health governance (ibid., p. 309). Although the empirical lineage of events outlined earlier in this book suggests that the IO was in fact quite late to adopt the health security discourse, Davies attributes the organization with having been complicit with this agenda, ostensibly to 'entrench' and increase 'its power to the point where it now presides over the global response to infectious disease outbreaks' (ibid., p. 312). Davies argues that in doing so, however, the WHO has compromised its moral authority so much so that it has potentially damaged its ability to assist developing countries respond to outbreaks (ibid., p. 296).

As noted above, the second source of overt criticism of the WHO has arisen from Hanrieder and Kreuder-Sonnen (2014). Attributing wide-sweeping powers of compulsion to the WHO secretariat, these authors argue that the IO utilized its newly endorsed emergency powers under the IHR (2005) to perpetrate a series of 'grave shortcomings' in its overall management of the 2009 H1N1 influenza pandemic (ibid., p. 12), even purportedly 'forcing' governments to inappropriately procure large stockpiles of influenza vaccines and antivirals via its declaration of a pandemic (ibid., p. 10). They subsequently go on to contend that the IO's new 'emergency powers are not only the products but also drivers of securitization' (ibid.), suggesting that there is an incentive for the WHO secretariat to declare further emergencies to justify their new authority, but they also argue for a series of additional oversight mechanisms to prevent future abuses of IO power.

Although Hanrieder and Kreuder-Sonnen's critique is subject to exaggeration and a limited understanding of the WHO's constitutional oversight mechanisms that are already in place,[1] their explicit criticism of the IO (and to a lesser extent Davies') is nonetheless somewhat rare amongst the scholarly community, prompting the question of why this is the case. Three conceivable explanations may be offered. The first possible reason is that both the public health and politics/IR scholars have unanimously concluded that the WHO is ultimately the sum of its parts with very little IO autonomy and that, accordingly, explicit criticism of the WHO secretariat's actions in securitizing certain health issues would be unjustified and unwarranted. Said another way, academe have acknowledged that the IO is subordinate to the directions and policy shifts of its principals, and given that the bulk of member states supported the health-as-security frame, the WHO secretariat was obliged to re-cast its public health mandate in security terms. Crucially, however, while it is accepted that a significant proportion of scholars working in this field may have engendered such a worldview, this explanation is arguably the least convincing as it discounts both the possibility of the WHO developing independent preferences that it may then seek to act upon (IO agency slack) as well as the prospect that the scholarly community holds divergent views and opinions.

The second, more plausible explanation is the influence that the WHO exerts. As noted in Chapter One, the WHO secretariat has at times been referred to as 'the medical mafia'. This descriptor, while usually used in the pejorative sense, nonetheless speaks to the composition of WHO employees, the majority of whom are medically trained professionals. These staff thereby form part of what could be described as a global epistemic community of health professionals – an epistemic community that, historically, has time and again been shown to be very reluctant to criticize its own members, usually due to a perceived professional courtesy. While this phenomenon may not necessarily extend to those on the outside of this community (namely to affect politics/IR scholars), many within the global public health community view the WHO as undertaking vitally important work and so could be reluctant to engage in overt criticism of the IO's actions. Fiona Godlee (2014), a well-known commentator on the WHO and now editor-in-chief of the *British Medical Journal*, has observed, for instance, that those who follow the WHO's work closely often possess an 'underlying loyalty to the concept. No one wants to see the organization disappear. Rather what it needs is adequate funds and strong leadership to do the job'. On the converse side, it has also been suggested that those who have criticized the WHO in the past have been intentionally prevented from gaining further access (Anonymous 2005), which suggests that some scholars may be reticent to admonish the IO due to concerns over perceived or actual retribution.

Equally, the work of Gagnon and Labonté (2013) alludes to a slightly different albeit related third possibility. In tracing the development of the United Kingdom's *Health is Global* white paper, which strongly promoted the health-as-security frame, the authors interviewed several officials that suggested that academic researchers had benefitted personally from 'piggybacking' onto the agenda (ibid., p. 6). As one interviewee characterized this trend:

> They (academic researchers) got invited to cabinet committees to sit at tables with four-star generals in a way that they weren't able to previously – academic researchers suddenly found that they could advocate for research funding because they were talking about things that might kill millions of people, like AIDS. (ibid., as quoted)

Another interviewee similarly observed, 'The security of health agenda has gone unchecked and unchallenged because too many people have too much to gain from it' (ibid., as quoted). While admittedly Gagnon and Labonté's research was limited to exploring the development of a national policy, it is equally reasonable to assume that a similar trend may have been replicated – at least to some degree – at the international level due to the prestige often associated with serving on international advisory panels such as the WHO expert committees. Accordingly, it may be that within some academic circles there is a practice of self-censorship underway to avoid the risk that it may jeopardize future professional standing.

The same concerns could not, however, be said to affect the IO's principals. As member states, even the organization's most distal principals have little to fear from the WHO secretariat, and this has been particularly reflected in the debates surrounding the IO's securitization of its public health mandate. In March 2007, for instance, prior to the official release of the 2007 World Health Report, the foreign affairs ministers of Brazil, France, Indonesia, Norway, Senegal, South Africa, and Thailand assembled in Oslo to discuss strategies to elevate health as a foreign policy issue. At the conclusion of the meeting these governments released what is now described as the 'Oslo Declaration', which outlined a series of 10 agenda items that included some 45 action points that would – theoretically – assist in raising health issues in international affairs. Yet despite the fact the very first agenda item was entitled 'Capacity for global health security', it was also observed that no consensus existed amongst the assembled foreign ministers as to what this phrase meant, and further elucidation would be sought at the next WHA (see Amorim et al. 2007).

Evidently, however, that illumination was not forthcoming. Indeed, within months of the release of the 2007 World Health Report that unambiguously announced the IO's adoption of the health-as-security frame, member states had assembled in Geneva, Switzerland, to commence negotiations on resolving a diplomatic impasse that had emerged following Indonesia's decision to cease sharing H5N1 virus samples with the GISN over a 'breakdown of mutual trust' (Sedyaningsih et al. 2008). The dispute highlighted the expanding disjuncture that was emerging between collective global health security and national security interests, for as attention increasingly focused on the 'global threat' from H5N1, member states moved to secure access to drug supplies to protect their respective populations. The outcome of this trend served to exacerbate the tensions between wealthier countries that could afford to enter into advance purchase agreements with pharmaceutical manufacturers to guarantee supply of these drugs and those countries that lacked the financial means to do so. The diplomatic quarrel arose when Indonesia then attempted to purchase influenza pharmaceuticals in late 2006 and was advised that it confronted a queue, even though samples provided by Indonesia to the WHO had been used to make the vaccines and the country was recording the highest number of human-related H5N1 deaths. In response, Indonesia announced that it would cease sharing H5N1 samples and called on the WHO to reform the influenza technical cooperation network to ensure that all participating countries gained equitable benefits. While condemned by a number of commentators from high-income countries claiming that the world was being held to ransom (Holbrooke and Garrett 2008), Indonesia's position found favour with a number of other low-income countries that confronted the same challenges.

The four-day meeting in November 2007 was thus the first official IGM to discuss the diplomatic impasse and try to develop a solution to address the concerns of Indonesia and like-minded countries. Throughout the meeting high-income countries, via a representative from the EU, attempted to pressure Indonesia into resuming its virus-sharing activities, citing that it was an obligation under the IHR (2005). Yet when the EU attempted to insert language on 'global health security' into the draft text on virus sharing, it prompted a 'heated controversy' before being rejected by a number of low- and middle-income countries that included Indonesia, India, Brazil, and Thailand (Sangeeta 2007, Tayob 2008). Ultimately it took a further three IGMs as well as an additional three IGWG meetings before consensus was finally reached – the 2011 PIP Framework that was endorsed by the 64th WHA on 2 May 2011. Significantly, no mention of 'global health security' or its derivatives were included.

In fact, disagreement over the WHO's adoption of the health-as-security frame escalated and was replicated in other forums, including the WHO's EB. At the 122nd EB in 2008 – the first EB meeting after the release of the 2007 World Health Report – the delegate from Brazil went to considerable lengths to stress that there was no consensus about the use of the phrase 'global health security' or its meaning (WHO EB 2008a). The representative further expressed Brazil's strong objection to the connections the WHO secretariat was making with the IHR (2005), and in particular the claim that the revised framework was 'an important instrument for ensuring that the goal of international public health security' was met (ibid., p. 58, see also Tayob 2008). As the representative later stated, the 2007 report included 'confrontational language that was more appropriate to the UN Security Council than to the International Health Regulations (2005)' (ibid., p. 151). While no objections were raised by other member states at that juncture, when the topic of climate change arose, Thailand also joined Brazil in condemning the use of the phrase 'global health security' (ibid., p. 67). As a consequence, while the resolution on climate change retained a reference to global health security, the EB resolution that was later passed on progressing the IHR's implementation made no mention of health security, at the global level or otherwise.[2]

Likewise, discord over the WHO secretariat's adoption of health-as-security additionally emerged and was reflected in discussions regarding the IO's official programme of work. Traditionally, every 10 years member states agree upon the overall strategy, priorities, and focus of the WHO's work for the coming decade. These 10-year strategic frameworks (otherwise referred to as the organization's 'General Programme of Work') then serve as the basis upon which medium-term six-year planning documents are developed, which in turn inform the IO's biannual funding and immediate assignments. In 2006, the 11th General Programme of Work 2006–2015 strategy document was released (WHO 2006e). This document, which was entitled 'Engaging for Health', made frequent reference to the WHO's global health security agenda and identified '[b]uilding individual and global health security' as the IO's second topmost category of work (ibid., see pp. ii, 14–15) (see also Table 6.1 for a full list of categories). Giving further weight to the importance of this objective, '[s]trengthening global health security' was acknowledged to be a key priority in the IO's medium-term strategic plan over the 2008–2013 period (ibid., p. iv).[3]

As a result of these declared priorities various country strategies were developed,[4] but in May 2013 member states again met in Geneva in the context of the 66th WHA to review the ongoing planning and development of the IO's 12th General Programme of Work (WHO 2013b). Some years on, the strategic document that outlines the WHO's future priorities remains in draft format; yet it is intriguing to note that at a meeting in February 2012 the IO's principals agreed that the organization's next programme of work would be arranged differently around five 'programmatic' areas – communicable diseases; non-communicable diseases; promoting health through the life-course; health systems; and preparedness, surveillance, and response – and a sixth work area pertaining to the IO's corporate services (ibid., p. 33) (see also Table 6.1). Even more intriguing was that with this change in direction the only reference to the concept of health security that was made in the first draft of the strategy document (submitted to the 65th WHA in May 2012) described the goal of 'collective security against health threats' (WHO 2012c, p. 9). No mention was made of the IO's mandate to ensure global health security, nor indeed did the phrase

Table 6.1 WHO work programme priorities

Categories	11th General Programme of Work	12th General Programme of Work (2013 Draft)	12th General Programme of Work
1	Investing in health to reduce poverty	Communicable diseases	Universal health coverage
2	Building individual and global health security	Non-communicable diseases	Millennium Development Goals
3	Promoting universal coverage, gender equality, and health-related human rights	Promoting health through the life-course	Non-communicable diseases
4	Tackling the determinants of health	Health systems	Implementing the International Health Regulations (2005)
5	Strengthening health systems and equitable access	Preparedness, surveillance, and response	Medical products
6	Harnessing knowledge, science, and technology	Corporate services	Social, economic, and environmental determinants of health
7	Strengthening governance, leadership, and accountability	—	

Sources: WHO (2006e); WHO (2013b); Cassels et al. (2014)

appear in any of the usual progress reports produced that year in relation to the implementation of the IHR (2005), pandemic preparedness, or the IO's role in humanitarian emergencies (see WHO 2012d, 2012e, 2012f).[5] Similarly, the phrase 'global health security' does not appear once in the 48-page draft document tendered at the 66th WHA, and only two references were made to 'health security' – once in relation to the IHR (2005), with the second appearing at the end of a statement of intent pertaining to preparedness, surveillance, and response (WHO 2014g, pp. 30, 33). Such omissions, while notable in light of the WHO secretariat's previous sponsorship of the global health security discourse, are not particularly surprising when also taking into account the discussions that transpired since 2011 regarding the WHO reform process.

Indeed, by 2009 the impact of the previous year's global financial crisis and the associated downturn of voluntary and assessed contributions was already being felt by a number of UN agencies, including the WHO (WHO EB 2010b, WHO 2010c, Leach-Kemon et al. 2012). The fiscal tightening subsequently led the WHO director-general to initiate an organization-wide review of its programmes and spending priorities, the findings of which were then tabled in a report and presented at the 128th EB in January 2011 (WHO EB 2010c),[6] ahead of the 64th WHA in May that same year (WHO 2011d). Following member states' deliberations, a new and extensive programme to reform the IO was given preliminary approval. Throughout 2011 a series of regional consultations were held with member states in which they examined the recommended streamlining of the WHO's core priorities and activities.

As recounted by the WHO secretariat in a series of reports submitted to a special session of the EB in November 2011, the majority of member states endorsed the overall recommendations and proposed direction for reforming the IO. Although the draft documentation that governments were supplied is not all publicly available, for the purposes of this book it can be ascertained from the secretariat reports that some adjustments had been made to the terminology regarding the WHO's core priorities. For example, whereas the IO's 11th General Programme of Work and the organization's 2008–2013 medium-term strategic plan had explicitly identified global health security as a core priority (see above), reflecting the concerns that had been previously raised by some member states, the WHO secretariat outlined yet another re-alignment to its overall approach for attaining the highest possible level of health for all peoples, advocating that five principles or 'pillars' of primary healthcare be used to inform its future activities (WHO EB 2011a, p. 3). As outlined in one of the reports, these included:

(a) reducing exclusion and social disparities in health;
(b) organizing health services around people's needs and expectations;
(c) integrating health into all sectors;
(d) pursuing collaborative models of policy dialogue; and
(e) increasing stakeholder participation. (ibid.)

To accomplish these objectives, the WHO secretariat proposed that the IO's activities be realigned around 'five core business areas' that were broadly described as: health systems and institutions, health development, health security, convening for better health, and evidence on health trends and determinants (ibid., pp. 3–4). As can be observed though, in describing these new foci all reference to 'global' was removed; and the references that were made to 'health security' (see also WHO EB 2011b, p. 5; 2011c, p. 3) sought to draw upon the definition that had been provided in May 2011 at the 64th WHA, which described the concept as:

> the strengthening of *national* and *international* capacity to reduce peoples' vulnerability to public health risks and to implement appropriate action when adverse events occur. Threats may arise from disease outbreaks such as cholera, pandemic influenza or SARS, or from physical causes such as radiation. Many threats are acute, but others are more long term (for instance, the impact of climate change or environmental pollution). Natural disasters, conflict and its aftermath pose similar challenges through their direct impact on individuals and the risks to health that arise from the disruption of essential services and the breakdown of state structures. (WHO 2011d, p. 8, emphasis added)

Even so, some member states still appeared dissatisfied with this compromise, stressing the need for the WHO secretariat to review the 'proposed core areas of work to determine whether they will respond in a manner that addresses the current needs of health systems' and to engage in 'further discussion based on a more in-depth analysis of the needs of the Member States' (WHO EB 2011c, pp. 5, 9). Yet other countries were even more explicit, arguing that 'more funds be channelled to areas that deal with non-communicable diseases, maternal and child health, and health systems, which [they] considered as being of overriding importance' (WHO EB 2011a, p. 5).

By 2014 it appeared that the WHO secretariat had almost entirely will-ingly jettisoned its utilization of the health-as-security discourse.[7] The one notable exception to this trend was the production of a report on antimicrobial resistance (AMR) that the secretariat published in April 2014 that identified 'AMR is a global health security threat that requires concerted cross-sectional action by governments and society as a whole' (WHO 2014i, p. xiii). Beyond this, as reflected in an article published by three senior WHO officials, Cassels, Smith, and Burci (Cassels et al. 2014), – global health security and any associated derivatives had been entirely removed from the WHO's priorities. Rather, the IO's key objec-tives were now identified as advancing universal health coverage, addressing current and future health-related MDGs, non-communicable diseases, implementing the IHR (2005), increasing access to medical products such as pharmaceutical and other health technologies, and addressing the social, economic, and environmental determinants of health (ibid., p. 203). Even in relation to the IHR, which had previously been frequently associated with the pursuit of global health security, the descriptors had reverted to expressing technocratic, technical terminol-ogy that would minimize the risk of antagonizing those member states dissatisfied with the health-as-security discourse.

It thus appears that the disgruntlement over the organization's pro-motion of global health security persisted amongst some of the IO's principals. No doubt concerned over the potential repercussions that might ensue if this issue was left unaddressed – such as the imposition of yet further economic, legal, or political mechanisms of control – the WHO secretariat capitulated to the small but vocal minority of member states by moderating its use of the health-as-security rhetoric. Indeed, as can be observed from the above analysis, since 2007 there has been a progressive winding back of the IO's global health security framing efforts, with the secretariat seeking to again re-cast its mandate and activities in a more technical, apolitical light. Such moves could be interpreted by some as the secretariat intentionally engaging in IO slip-page; and yet the converse argument could also be made that the WHO is rather responding to the expressed preferences of its member states and dutifully following their directions. Certainly, given that consensus evidently does not exist, the IO has sought to distance itself from the health-as-security discourse and thereby circumvent any disruption to its activities. In the remainder of this chapter, the implications of these moves and counter-moves will be examined in greater detail, with par-ticular attention given to the impact on the role and function of the WHO's disease eradication mandate. In this, recent history may offer an indication of what is to come.

So, what happens now?

There is little question that the securitization of health issues perpetrated over the past few decades has yielded considerable benefits. Indeed, even the staunchest critics of the health-as-security discourse have acknowledged the advantages that securitization brings in the form of heightened political awareness and engagement, which in turn frequently leads to the allocation of significant financial resources to address the perceived threat (see, for example, Ingram 2005, Collier and Lakoff 2008, Abraham 2011). In this regard, the successful securitization of specific health issues such as pandemic influenza, HIV/AIDS, and biological weapons substantiates the notable benefits that can accrue. Leaving aside for a moment whether in fact the connections that have been efficaciously drawn between acute hazards to human health and national/international security can now be 'un-made' (see Concluding Remarks), the desecuritization of health issues is likely to have a deleterious impact – at least to some extent – on the WHO's disease eradication mandate.

The framing of certain health issues in security terms actively contributed to health being recognized as a legitimate foreign policy issue (McInnes and Lee 2006). High-income countries the world over subsequently recognized that by assisting their less wealthy compatriots to improve their disease surveillance capacities and health systems, they in turn would help themselves by decreasing the risk of diseases spreading to their territories and respective populations. This oft-repeated refrain that diseases do not respect human-imposed borders and enlightened self-interest proved to be a powerful motivating force, encouraging governments to look for ways and means to aid low- and middle-income countries build and strengthen their health infrastructure. It has been in this context that the WHO has benefitted tremendously for a time from high-income countries' anxieties, as Davies (2008) accurately identifies in her critique. For while the field of global health has become increasingly crowded with the influx of multiple new actors, the WHO has continued to retain its overall reputation as the world's leading technical agency in international health matters.

Said another way, particularly since the start of the new millennium there has been a direct correlation between the level of financial and political support that the WHO has received and the securitization of health issues. That the WHO secretariat would have collectively recognized this phenomenon and subsequently further encouraged its development through the release of policy documents and key publications in academic journals is entirely consistent with most theories of IO pathology, and thus should come as no particular surprise. Accordingly, while some critics may seek to suggest that the organization's activities simply reflected the interests of the most powerful and influential (proximal) member states, implying that the WHO is merely a puppet whose strings are being pulled, it is equally plausible that this was one instance where the collective preferences of the IO and the vast majority of its masters aligned closely, if not entirely. It is also in this same regard, however, that in the event the WHO secretariat seeks to now distance itself too much from the health-as-security discourse, there will likely be financial and political repercussions.

It is important to recall, for instance, that there have been unprecedented levels of growth in official development assistance (ODA) and non-governmental funding for health over the past few decades. Between 1990 and 1997, ODA and non-governmental funding grew by 49 per cent, from US$5.74 billion to US$8.54 billion. Between 1998 and 2012, however, ODA and non-governmental funding such as philanthropic donations for health increased by over 230 per cent to peak in 2012 at US$28.2 billion (IHME 2012, Lidén 2014). While a substantial proportion of this growth can be attributed to other factors such as the creation of the MDGs and associated global health partnerships like the Global Fund to Fight AIDS, TB, and Malaria, it has to be equally acknowledged that the securitization of specific acute health hazards provided additional impetus for high-income countries to significantly increase financial contributions.

For the WHO, while the organization's biannual budget more than doubled over the 10-year period from US$1.6 billion in 1998–1999 to US$4.2 billion in 2008–2009 (Sridhar and Gostin 2011), the vast majority of these increases were provided in the form of extrabudgetary voluntary contributions. In 1998–1999, for instance, voluntary contributions rested at approximately 48 per cent of the IO's total funds (ibid.), but by 2010–2011 75 per cent of the WHO's programmes were funded by extrabudgetary funds, and some 91 per cent of these monies were reserved for specific donor-driven priorities (van de Pas and van Schaik 2014, p. 197). Earmarked extrabudgetary funds later increased to a total of 77 per cent of the IO's funding arrangements in 2014–2015 (Gautier et al. 2014, pp. 172, 177). Equally significant for the purposes of this book, between 2008 and 2009 approximately 60 per cent of the IO's extrabudgetary funds were allocated explicitly for the prevention and control of infectious disease (Sridhar and Gostin 2011, p. 1586), and this overall trend has continued (see Sridhar et al. 2014).

Even taking into account the criticisms that have emerged post-2007, therefore, it remains highly improbable that the WHO secretariat would suddenly announce to the international community that it was no longer prepared to describe its disease eradication mandate in security terms. Such a course of action would have little benefit, as it would be unlikely to assuage the concerns of its critics while simultaneously risking that member states would reallocate extrabudgetary funds to other organizations. Further, such a path would be unwise, particularly given that the majority of member states continue to appear reasonably comfortable with the concept and its use. Throughout various EB meetings, for instance, governments as diverse as Chile, Kuwait, Lithuania, Morocco, the People's Republic of China, Somalia, and the Syrian Arab Republic have indicated their support of the WHO's use of global health security by adopting its terminology to advocate for particular programmes or policies (WHO EB 2010a, p. 96; 2011d, p. 129; 2012, pp. 144–153; 2013, pp. 140–146). These governments thus join others that include Australia, Switzerland, the United States, and the 28 members of the EU that have consistently supported the health-as-security frame (WHO EB 2011d, pp. 132–134; 2013, pp. 142–146).

Moreover, in what must be an especially perplexing situation for the IO some member states have exhibited inconsistency towards this issue. For example, in 2007 Sri Lanka observed that 'one of the Secretariat's functions was to provide technical expertise to Member States in order to ensure global health security' (WHO EB 2007, p. 111), yet in 2011 the same government was calling for more clarity on the concept and discouraging its use (WHO EB 2011d, p. 134). Likewise, in 2007 Thailand and Indonesia indicated their solidarity with Brazil in questioning the WHO's use of the phrase 'global health security' (Sangeeta 2007). Yet in 2009 Indonesia engaged the same terminology to push for a resolution to the Israel–Palestine conflict as well as advocate for more resources to strengthen health systems (WHO EB 2009, pp. 58, 77), whereas Thailand even went so far as to state in 2013, following the adoption of the 2011 PIP Framework, 'The Secretariat should continue its efforts to increase the influenza vaccine supply in the interests of global health security. Legal complexities should not be allowed to block the global health security movement' (WHO EB 2013, p. 147).

It can be clearly observed, therefore, that there is still considerable ambiguity amongst the WHO's principals as to the benefit and utility of the health-as-security discourse. However, where some might anticipate that the WHO secretariat would take advantage of this equivocality to drive forward its own agenda, intentionally engaging in agency slack, the IO has instead quietly reversed course. In fact, to date the route that the WHO secretariat appears to have adopted following the criticisms that emerged from 2007 onwards has been to downplay the health-as-security frame, which it has done by simply avoiding it and selecting instead to re-cast the activities previously described as essential to global health security – such as the IHR (2005) – in technocratic language.

The ultimate outcome of the WHO secretariat's decision to reframe its disease eradication mandate and activities in more conventional public health terminology remains to be seen. Given the role that securitization had though in elevating health as a legitimate foreign policy issue at the turn of the new millennium, it can be anticipated that the IO's unwillingness to now utilize and promote its health-as-security mandate may result in some unintended consequences. Arguably, however, here the greatest risk is to the WHO.

There is a genuine possibility, for instance, that by actively suppressing the health-as-security discourse, some member states – and particularly the IO's proximal principals that have been very supportive of this agenda – will interpret this move as the WHO shirking its delegated responsibilities. Were this to occur, it is likely that they would again begin to question the IO's continued relevance in a manner consistent with the events of 1994 that prompted the creation of UNAIDS. Although somewhat speculative, a close reading of the speeches delivered by Director-General Margaret Chan after the WHO reform process was launched in 2010 reveals that at least some elements of the secretariat appear to be acutely aware of the risk to the organization's reputation.

In 2011, for example, in a speech delivered at the EB special session on WHO reform, the director-general observed, 'These are issues where our reputation stands or falls depending on how nimble and capable we are in addressing these challenges or paving the path for others to do so' (WHO EB 2011e, p. 1). The issues that Dr Chan was referring to included the five 'flagship' reform priorities that had been collectively agreed by member states and which notably included (at that time) health security. The director-general went on to state:

> WHO made much of its reputation fighting infectious diseases, bringing many to their knees. Rest assured: we will never let down our guard. We know how quickly infectious diseases, even when apparently close to control, can take advantage of any opportunity to resurge with a vengeance. (ibid.)

In making this speech, which occurred even as the WHO secretariat was censoring its use of 'global health security' throughout various policy documents and reports, the director-general sought to highlight that while the IO's rhetoric had altered, in reality its practices would not dramatically change. Additional speeches delivered by the WHO director-general from 2012 to 2014 further corroborate this conclusion.

As noted earlier, the WHO secretariat has frequently pronounced the IHR (2005), and in particular real-time disease surveillance, as fundamental to global health security. Addressing the 65th WHA in May 2012 the director-general remarked in her opening speech that progress continued apace in implementing the IHR core capacities, due to the IO's 'sophisticated electronic surveillance system' that gathered disease intelligence in real-time. The director-general further stated, 'We are rarely taken by surprise. WHO can mount an international response within 24 hours . . . No other agency can do this' (WHO 2012g, p. 3). The following year, in responding to member states' interventions at the 66th WHA regarding progress in implementing the IHR (2005), the director-general underlined that the WHO's coordination role under the revised framework was 'essential' due to the fact that 'a coordination mechanism was required in order to bring together the world's assets and determine whether any new pathogen would pose a public health risk of international concern' (WHO 2013c, p. 12). The IHR (2005), which the director-general then described as 'a legal framework for strengthening the global defence system against new and emerging infectious diseases' (ibid.), needed urgent funding though, to ensure that the IO's effectiveness and assistance to countries was not compromised.

Similarly, the growing prevalence of AMR is an issue that had been previously identified by the WHO as a direct concern to global health security (see Hardiman 2003, WHO 2007a, p. xi). National governments such as the United Kingdom, Sweden, and the United States have likewise explicitly described increasing resistance as a threat to global health security and advocated global action (WHO 2013d, Gostin and Phelan 2014). Yet in her opening speech to the 67th WHA in 2014, while no reference to global health security was made, the WHO director-general stressed that:

> We learned, too, how much the world needs an organization like WHO. Within the framework of our leadership priorities, WHO is shaping the health agenda as needs evolve, and using multiple mechanisms and partnerships to meet these needs. If anything, the relevance of this Organization has increased . . . WHO constantly

monitors evolving trends and sounds the alarm when needed. For communicable diseases, one of the most alarming crises is the rise of antimicrobial resistance, which WHO documented in a report last month. This is a crisis that now affects every region of the world, and it is only getting worse. (WHO 2014g)

These statements reflect the ongoing petition by the WHO secretariat to member states that the organization remains committed to fulfilling its delegated responsibilities, even though the discourse surrounding the IO's disease eradication mandate may have been reworked again. It is also in this regard, however, that the changes to the WHO's delegation contract that were instituted by member states while revising the IHR may prove to be the most significant challenge for the IO.

As outlined in Chapter Four, several adjustments were made to the WHO's disease eradication delegation contract throughout the process of the IHR IGWG that have affected the manner in which the IO fulfils its duties. While some elements of the WHO's new approach to managing global health security were enshrined and protected under the revised IHR framework, such as the IO's ability to utilize non-government sources of information to identify disease outbreaks and the ability to 'name and shame' governments, equally member states moved decisively to circumvent the WHO secretariat possessing too much autonomy that might adversely impact state sovereignty. New legislative control mechanisms were inserted that place procedural limitations on the WHO secretariat unilaterally declaring a PHEIC, and member states also clarified the types of recommendations they believed the IO was best qualified to issue.

In the context of the 2009 H1N1 influenza pandemic, the WHO secretariat appeared to function well even with these new constraints, and its management of the event was not – at least at first glance – unduly compromised. No doubt the new requirement for the director-general to convene and consult with the IHR Emergency Committee prior to making any notable decisions proved at times to be frustrating for elements of the secretariat that wanted rapid and decisive action to halt the spread of the virus. But equally, in another sense the IHR Emergency Committee proved to be an important shield for the WHO director-general against criticisms that later arose, as her decisions and determinations were backed by an independent expert panel. Likewise, the WHO secretariat's ability to issue recommendations and policy advice in real-time was not especially curtailed. Throughout the pandemic the IO was observed to constantly update the information and advice it was providing, issue new case definitions and advice on treatment, and recommend measures that governments could take to help reduce the number of infections.

Having said this, it is clear that in other respects the WHO secretariat was overly cautious to avoid the risk of antagonizing its member states. This was most clearly observed in relation to the IO's evident lack of willingness to criticize those governments that imposed temporary travel restrictions on Mexican and North American citizens (irrespective of whether or not they had been at risk of physical exposure), applied trade import bans on pork and pork products (even though there was no evidence to suggest a risk of transmission), and decimated pig populations for no other stated reason than to assuage public fear. In practice, therefore, the WHO secretariat – and particularly the director-general – resiled from its role as government assessor and critic that it had performed throughout the 2003 SARS outbreak, presumably because it was concerned that such actions may result in the IO being subjected to new political, legislative, or financial constraints.

In defence of the WHO, it could be argued that the 2009 H1N1 pandemic was the first test of the revised IHR framework, and so the organization was in the process of ascertaining the boundaries of its newly revised authority. Although such an assertion largely ignores the precedents established by the IO's successful management of the 2003 SARS outbreak, it would be reasonable in this context to allow the organization further opportunity to demonstrate how it would fulfil its updated mandate. Even in this respect though, the WHO secretariat did not have long to wait before further opportunities presented themselves in the form of yet another novel coronavirus and an unprecedented outbreak of EVD.

In late September 2012, authorities in the United Kingdom informed the WHO secretariat that a new coronavirus had been detected in a patient transferred from Qatar. The pathogen responsible had already been isolated by a clinic in The Netherlands following a previous fatality in Saudi Arabia, so this second case raised concerns that a new, albeit small outbreak may be underway (WHO 2013e). In response, the WHO secretariat encouraged governments throughout the region and beyond to undertake increased surveillance; over the coming months, further isolated cases were identified across a number of Middle Eastern countries. By 23 May 2013 the IO had received reports of 44 confirmed cases that included 22 fatalities throughout Jordan, Qatar, Saudi Arabia, and the United Arab Emirates, but cases had also been detected in France, Germany, Tunisia, and the United Kingdom (WHO 2013f). The extent of the outbreak subsequently prompted an expert panel to give the new disease a name – the Middle East Respiratory Syndrome (MERS-CoV) (WHO 2013g).

In many respects, the WHO's management of the MERS-CoV outbreak initially replicated many of the organization's now-standard functions. Immediately upon receipt of the UK authorities' report, for example, the WHO secretariat instigated its real-time epidemic intelligence coordinator role by collecting data on confirmed and suspected cases, as well as information on the measures governments were taking to treat patients. This information was then collated and analysed to inform the WHO's recommendations, which were constantly revised and updated as new information came to light (WHO 2013h).[8] In an attempt to avoid a repeat of measures taken throughout the 2009 H1N1 influenza pandemic, guidelines based on available evidence were produced and disseminated on various related topics such as infection control, technical assistance was rendered (WHO 2014h), and advice was issued with virtually every update that screening at airports was unnecessary and that trade and travel restrictions were unwarranted.

Nonetheless, by July 2013 the number of cases had continued to progressively grow, indicating that the outbreak was far from controlled. Confronted with some 80 laboratory-confirmed cases and 44 deaths (WHO 2013i), the director-general invoked the IHR (2005) for a second time and convened the IHR Emergency Committee, which met for the first time on 9 July 2013 (WHO 2013j). Citing a lack of sufficient information, the Committee reconvened via teleconference a week later on 17 July (and, at least at the time of writing, has met an additional five times) to review the epidemiological situation and make a determination on whether the conditions to declare a PHEIC had been met. At the emergency committee's seventh meeting on 1 October 2014 the expert panel again confirmed that as there was no evidence of sustained human-to-human transmission and that, accordingly, while continued vigilance was deemed essential, declaration of a PHEIC was not justified (WHO 2014j).

Even from the brief summary provided above, it can be observed that the WHO's management of the MERS-inspired public health crisis is very different from the organization's response to SARS. From an epidemiological standpoint there are very good reasons for this, none the least because unlike SARS the MERS-CoV pathogen has yet to achieve the ability to transmit readily between humans. Were this to change, it can be anticipated that the IO's response to the disease – not to mention member states' – would alter dramatically. Even so, it is clear that the

WHO has approached the management of this new health hazard in a very orderly manner, ensuring that it has fully complied with the procedural requirements under the revised IHR (2005) to consult with all relevant parties affected by the disease prior to issuing advice and recommending how governments respond. Furthermore, in reviewing various statements made by senior members of the WHO secretariat, it is also apparent that the additional checks and balances instituted by member states throughout the IHR revision process has made the IO even more cautious in its approach.

For example, at the 66th WHA on 23 May 2013 the WHO secretariat and Saudi Arabia's Ministry of Health arranged a special presentation on MERS-CoV for the assembled government representatives. At the briefing, Saudi Arabia's Deputy Minister for Health, Dr Z. A. Memish, identified that one of the key challenges his country and other affected countries encountered in controlling the virus' spread was the inability to develop an effective diagnostic test. This situation had arisen though, Dr Memish relayed, as a direct consequence of a laboratory in The Netherlands that had chosen to patent the virus and sign a contract with a pharmaceutical manufacturer that restricted access to the pathogen for other research laboratories without a strict legal agreement in place (otherwise known as 'material transfer agreements') (WHO 2013k). Yet, despite the fact that Dr Keiji Fukuda, WHO Assistant Director-General for the Health Security and Environment Cluster, and WHO Director-General Chan publicly urged member states to ensure that intellectual property considerations should not be permitted to adversely affect public health (ibid., p. 13), no additional criticisms – either of the laboratory, the pharmaceutical manufacturer, or of the countries in which these organizations were based – were made. Similarly, when questioned the following day over the fact that the WHO secretariat had failed to issue any travel advisories for affected countries, particularly in light of the upcoming hajj in Saudi Arabia, Dr Fukuda responded by noting that 'making such recommendations was one of the Secretariat's most difficult tasks' (WHO 2013c, p. 11). Dr Fukuda went on to observe that while he and his staff wanted to ensure that all necessary steps were taken to prevent the pathogen's further spread, they 'also recognized that travel was the lifeblood of many countries' (ibid.).

These comments are remarkable because they indicate that the WHO secretariat has become far more circumspect in how it carries out its disease eradication delegation contract, apparently even in relation to the actions allegedly perpetrated by non-state actors. It will be recalled, for instance, that the Chinese government's actions in 2003 in attempting to hide the true nature of their SARS epidemic provoked a sharp rebuke from WHO Director-General Brundtland and several senior members of her staff. While some speculated after the event that the director-general was so critical only because she was not seeking re-election for a second term (Anonymous 2005), Dr Brundtland maintained that her actions were based on a 'lifetime of experience' and that the organization had responded appropriately 'given its mandate' (Brundtland 2006). More than a decade later, however, after the IHR revision and in the wake of the IO being accused of being inappropriately influenced by commercial interests into declaring a pandemic, the WHO secretariat finds itself in a more tightly controlled and regulated environment.

It is in this regard that the above comments also suggest that the measures instituted by member states to limit the IO's autonomy have proved largely successful, not only in ensuring that the WHO secretariat is prevented from taking unilateral action (such as declaring a PHEIC) but also in guaranteeing that the IO consults far more closely and regularly with countries prior to issuing recommendations. At the same time, in the specific context of MERS-CoV, it does not appear that the new procedures the WHO secretariat is required to follow have unduly hampered its management of the crisis; but as noted earlier, epidemiologically MERS-CoV is currently a very different pathogen from SARS or a novel influenza strain. Regrettably, the extent of the IO's new measured, guarded approach to managing global health security is also now being firmly tested in the context of a fast-moving and virulent health hazard – EVD.

At the time of writing, the international community is confronted with an unprecedented outbreak of Ebola in West Africa that has already resulted in more than 21,700 people infected and over 8,600 deaths. This outbreak, which is already the largest in recorded human history, originally began on 26 December 2013 in a remote border region between Guinea, Liberia, and Sierra Leone (WHO 2014k), but remained largely undetected for almost three months until the ministry of health in Guinea reported to the WHO a total of 49 cases and 29 fatalities on 23 March 2014 (WHO 2014l). Within a week, the Liberian and Sierra Leonean health authorities reported additional cases (WHO 2014m, 2014n), and over the coming weeks the virus continued to spread before eventually appearing in Nigeria, Senegal, and the United States.[9] Upon receiving notification of the outbreak, utilizing GOARN, the WHO assembled and dispatched foreign medical teams to assist local health authorities. Médecins Sans Frontières (MSF), which already had personnel in-country assisting with a malaria outbreak, responded by establishing healthcare facilities in affected areas (WHO 2014k). As the weeks progressed though, the number of infected persons seeking care overwhelmed MSF's resources, and so in an attempt to garner more awareness of the unfolding humanitarian crisis and obtain additional help, the NGO began issuing press releases calling for international assistance.

To a large extent, however, the calls from MSF went unheeded by the WHO and the wider international community until September 2014.[10] On 7 and 8 August, in response to reports that Ebola cases had begun to appear in neighbouring Nigeria, the WHO director-general convened the IHR Emergency Committee via teleconference (WHO 2014o). The committee unanimously agreed that a PHEIC was underway, and urged those countries affected to declare a state of national emergency and implement disaster management plans, while all other countries were encouraged to increase surveillance. The committee also recommended that travel restrictions should not be imposed on affected countries, reportedly in recognition that it would harm international relief efforts. Yet in a rather questionable decision, the IHR Emergency Committee did not call for international assistance to help contain the outbreak and recommended that the situation only be reviewed again in three months' time (ibid.).

By late August 2014 the outbreak had resulted in over 3,000 infections and 1,500 deaths (WHO 2014p). Overwhelmed, and in an extraordinary move for the NGO, on 2 September 2014 MSF called for military intervention to help contain the outbreak (Hussain 2014), even as senior UN leaders were gathering in Washington, DC to discuss how to escalate international assistance in light of the growing humanitarian crisis (WHO 2014r). On 16 September 2014 President Obama announced his country's commitment to deploy 3,000 military personnel to West Africa to help construct Ebola treatment facilities and train local health workers (Mason and Giahyue 2014). This commitment, which in early October was expanded to potentially 4,000 personnel (Stewart 2014), was replicated on a smaller scale by other governments deploying military forces to aid containment efforts, including the United Kingdom, France, Germany, and eventually China. Importantly, however, on 18 September the UN Security Council passed resolution 2177 (2014) declaring the Ebola outbreak 'a threat to international peace and security' (UN 2014b). At the same time, the UN established the first-ever public health mission: the United Nations Mission for Ebola Emergency Response (UNMEER).

The passage of resolution 2177(2014) and the creation of UNMEER has been interpreted as a stunning indictment of the WHO's failure in responding to the EVD crisis (Fidler 2014). Public criticisms of the WHO's handling of the Ebola outbreak began to emerge from July 2014 onwards[11] and ranged from the delay taken in convening the IHR Emergency Committee, to 'a culture of stagnation' (Gostin, cited in Gale and Lauerman 2014), to the dysfunctional relationship between the central headquarters and the African regional office. In mid-October 2014 an internal document was leaked to the world's media in which the WHO acknowledged that several factors had contributed to its mis-management of the outbreak, including serious incompetence (Cheng 2014). In response to the unexpected disclosure, the WHO released its own statement on 18 October, stressing that the report had not been 'fact-checked' and that 'A full review and analysis of global responses to this, the largest-ever Ebola outbreak in history, will be completed and made public once the outbreak is under control' (WHO 2014q).

There is little question that the WHO's handling of the Ebola outbreak in West Africa will be scrutinized extensively in the months and years to follow. Although some commentators have attempted to support the WHO, noting how the organization has been subject to extensive budget cuts that have hampered its operational response capabilities (see Fink 2014a), equally the failure of the IO to fulfil its health-as-security delega-tion contract will be viewed poorly by proximal and distal principals alike. One small indication of the level of member state dissatisfaction has already materialized with the replacement of the African regional office's director in November 2014 (AFRO 2014), but it is unlikely the political ramifications will cease there. Certainly the content of the internal report has confirmed what many critics have highlighted for years regarding the dissected nature of the WHO into effectively seven independent entities, and the ineptitude and duplication this structure creates.

Having said this, in the opening months of the 2014 West African Ebola outbreak the WHO was observed to institute its now-standard approach to global health security, fulfilling a number of roles in real-time wherever possible. For example, the IO continued to collect epide-miological intelligence and convert this information into policy-relevant advice as soon as information was reported to the WHO. Whereas the timeliness of the data and advice was perhaps not as 'real-time' as during previous outbreaks, some of the delays that were experienced can equally be attributed to the poor health infrastructure within the affected West African countries. In addition, the WHO facilitated the deployment of expert teams to assist countries with instituting containment measures, but when queried by a *New York Times* reporter in early September 2014, WHO Director-General Margaret Chan stressed, 'we are not the first responder. You know, the government has first priority to take care of their people and provide healthcare. W.H.O. is a technical agency' that did not provide 'direct services' (Fink 2014b).

The lack of direct action and leadership displayed by the WHO throughout the opening months of the EVD crisis was indubitably one of the key reasons for the creation of UNMEER. However, given that the WHO has consistently emphasized its ability to manage global health security since 2001, its incompetence within the context of the 2014 Ebola outbreak to assist governments contain the disease in a timely manner – either by providing resources in the initial weeks or raising the alarm sufficiently to rapidly assemble an international coalition – will reflect very negatively upon the IO's reputation. At the time of writing, UNMEER had been established for less than a few months, but it has already demonstrated the leadership that many in the international community would have been expecting to see emerge from the WHO. UNMEER has, for example, led the campaign for the quarantine and isolation of potential cases and the safe burials of victims within a 60-day timeframe (World Bank 2014). It has also coordinated the multiple UN agencies and non-government and civil society organizations now engaged within those countries affected by Ebola. While the health targets were developed in collaboration with the WHO and the IO continues to play a key technical role (UN 2014c), it was the Head of UNMEER, Anthony Banbury, who had exhibited leadership, assumed responsibility for coordinating the international response, and been consistently calling for more resources and personnel to fight Ebola, even as the WHO and its director-general have been eerily absent.

While the humanitarian crisis continues unabated there will be little time allocated to apportioning blame, as all partners are appropriately focused on containing this outbreak and saving lives. In the aftermath though, it can be anticipated that several investigations will be launched into the WHO's handling of the 2014 West African Ebola outbreak and the actions of the organization's secretariat. It is only then, perhaps, that some of the details as to why the IO has failed so spectacularly to fulfil its delegation contract and mandate in this context will emerge. Given the leaked internal report, attention will understandably focus on the relationship between the African regional office and the central head-quarters in Geneva, but questions as to why it took so long to convene the IHR Emergency Committee, and why its second meeting was only convened days after the UN Security Council resolution was passed, will be lines of inquiry that must be pursued. If member states are also consistent with past behaviour, it can be expected that in successive WHA meetings they will seek to impose additional control mechanisms on the WHO secretariat in the wake of the EVD crisis. Exactly what form those mechanisms may take – politico-legal, economic, technical, or socio-legal – is unclear, but it is improbable that the IO will escape unscathed.

Equally though, not all the blame can be attributed solely to the WHO and its regional office. In many respects, member states – and particularly some of the IO's proximal principals – must conceivably accept some of the blame for the WHO's mishandling of this latest PHEIC. It must be recalled, for instance, that the division of the WHO into seven organizations was the result of an historical anomaly whereby the Americas' regional office pointedly refused to be subsumed into the new universal health agency. The PASB/PAHO intransigence on this matter, and its insistence on no small measure of autonomy to decide upon its priorities and budgetary expenditure, set the precedent for the remaining regional structure of the IO. Added to this, the budget cuts that the organization has been subjected to via the WHO reform process of recent years have been extensive, and have been openly acknowledged to have caused staff reductions and the cancellation of programmes. As also explored in Chapter Four, following the 2003 SARS outbreak member states went to considerable lengths to convey to the secretariat that there are limits to the IO's autonomy that they are prepared to accept – a message that has evidently been heard by the organization's director-general and senior staff. While, therefore, mistakes and even IO slippage may have transpired in the Ebola response, the mismanagement of the crisis in the initial months and the dysfunction that ensued should have perhaps been anticipated, given the economic and politico-legal constraints that member states had previously imposed. Although it is dubious that member states will accept any responsibility for the IO's actions, what is apparent is that the WHO's management of the 2014 Ebola outbreak will likely feature prominently in providing new interpretations of the IO's authority both now and in the foreseeable future.

Conclusion

It took some years, but following the WHO secretariat's decision to reframe its public health mandate in security terms, a number of criticisms have emerged. As this chapter has shown, the critiques surfaced from two primary groups that included the academic community and a small but vocal number of member states. Even so, for almost a decade the WHO secretariat largely avoided being directly censured for its actions in promoting the securitization of certain select health issues, with much of the blame being attributed to powerful Western interests pressuring the WHO behind the scenes. While there may initially have been some validity to these claims, equally certain elements of the WHO secretariat (including its senior leadership) embraced the concept of global health security and utilized the health-as-security frame to successfully lobby for new powers and financial support to fulfil the organization's disease eradication delegation contract.

Nonetheless, in a move that would surprise many who view IOs as self-seeking aggrandizers, when criticisms later did emerge of the WHO's securitization efforts, rather than take advantage of member states' indecision the IO quietly and systematically initiated a process to reframe its activities again in a discourse more congenial to its disgruntled principals. In so doing though, the WHO now conceivably confronts a dangerous predicament whereby it risks being accused of shirking its delegated responsibilities by those member states that are supportive of the health-as-security agenda. While the agent continues to stress that it is only the rhetoric that may have changed, the WHO secretariat is also contending with new procedural measures designed to limit its autonomy in responding to disease outbreaks and, as recent events have revealed, these control mechanisms are having a demonstrable impact on the IO's performance. The future of the WHO's approach to managing global health security is thus again under question, and it is to this topic that the conclusion to this book now turns.

Concluding Remarks

Achieving good health is a constant struggle and, as this book's survey of the WHO's activities reveals, it is made no less difficult at the global level. Since the organization's creation in 1948 the WHO secretariat has adopted a number of methods and approaches to fulfil its overriding mandate to assist the attainment of the highest possible level of health for all peoples. The eradication of disease – particularly the infectious kind – is fundamental to that objective, existing as the precondition to the WHO's definition of health. Further reflecting the importance of this central mission, the IO's founders imbued the organization with considerable authority and autonomy to affect its disease eradication mandate. Over the years the WHO secretariat has sought to accomplish this assigned task by instituting a series of global disease eradication campaigns and establishing multiple disease eradication and/or control programmes. The lessons that the IO – and particularly its senior leadership – learned from these campaigns subsequently informed the organization's classical approach to disease eradication. Yet as the world continued to change and globalize, and member states continued to shirk their responsibilities in reporting disease outbreaks, the WHO was forced to adapt its methods and approach.

It is in this regard that the WHO's utilization of the health security discourse to reframe its public health mandate reflects yet another step in the IO's attempts to fulfil its delegated responsibilities. Like the organization's previous endeavours to use human rights, economic, and development arguments before it, the WHO secretariat has arguably used the concept of security to great effect, not only in securing new political attention and resources but also in obtaining additional powers. Following the WHO's successful management of the 2003 SARS outbreak, the IO also witnessed the further expansion of its authority, with several policies and procedures that had proved so effective in containing and eliminating the pathogen enshrined in another core element of the organization's delegation contract – the IHR (2005). Importantly, however, member states also revealed that they held concerns about the level and extent of IO autonomy that the organization had wielded throughout the SARS crisis, and so, using the vehicle of the IHR revision process, instituted several new legal and procedural mechanisms of control.

It took a number of years, but criticisms of the WHO secretariat's decision to securitize its public health mandate did also eventually emerge. While the IO could, and predictably has, largely ignored the denunciations arising from one group of detractors (namely elements of the academic community), as an intergovernmental organization answerable to its principals, the WHO has not been able to side-step the concerns raised by a small sub-set of member states quite so readily. In response to this latter group's concerns, the IO's secretariat has chosen to progressively desecuritize its disease eradication responsibilities by intentionally removing security-related language and concepts from policy documents, reports, and speeches. Somewhat surprisingly, the WHO secretariat has taken these actions despite the fact that, when collectively viewed, member states have continued to display considerable preference heterogeneity over this matter.

It therefore does not appear that the WHO can – at least in this instance – be accused of agency slack per se. In fact rather the opposite may be true. For while some governments that have been strong supporters of the health-as-security discourse may be tempted to suggest that the IO is currently engaging in a form of slippage, it could well be argued on the converse side that by removing virtually all reference to global health security the WHO secretariat's actions reflect significant sensitivity to its principals, even those who perhaps might otherwise be described as some of its more distal members. Importantly, however, in perpetrating this action, the WHO secretariat is also enacting a particular form of desecuritization.

According to the Copenhagen School's founders, securitization actually represents a breakdown of normal public policy processes to adequately deal with issues. Security, as Buzan et al. (1998, p. 29) observe, 'should be seen as negative, as a failure to deal with issues as normal politics'. This is principally because security 'works to silence opposition and has given power holders many opportunities to exploit "threats" for domestic purposes, to claim a right to handle something with less democratic control and constraint' (ibid.). In practice, therefore, Buzan and his colleagues contend that securitizing an issue elevates it and places it above standard political contestation and debate – what is described as 'hyper-politicization' – primarily as solutions are required as soon as possible to deal with the imminent 'threat'. Buzan et al. accept that some issues warrant this hyper-politicization, but maintain that ultimately the preferred option should be to reintegrate securitized issues into mainstream political bargaining processes and policy contestation. This process has been described as desecuritization, and remains at the normative heart of the Copenhagen School project.

Despite the fact that desecuritization serves as the definitive, preferred endpoint, to date very little of the security studies literature has actually attempted to engage with this concept, let alone how to achieve it. Generations of scholars have instead sought to dissect in ever-diminishing circles the core elements and minutiae of securitization theory, ranging from those fascinated with the process or outcomes of securitization and the roles and performativity of actors, moves, and audiences (Vuori 2008, Léonard and Kaunert 2011, Roe 2012), to those seeking to draw distinctions between 'internalist' and 'externalist' readings (Stritzel 2007), while yet others interrogate the theoretical, philosophical, sociological, or emancipatory potentialities of the theory (Williams 2003, Aradau 2004, Balzacq 2011, Nunes 2014). By way of comparison, very few scholars have engaged with how to affect desecuritization.

Having said this, the field is not completely devoid (see, for example, Wæver 1995, Knudsen 2001, Williams 2003, Aradau 2004, Roe 2004, MacKenzie 2009, McDonald 2011). In her work, Hansen (2012) has traced the existing theoretical and empirical pathways that actors have used to desecuritize certain issues, identifying that there have been four forms or categories that have been deployed to date. These categories have been described as: *change through stabilization*, which is when an issue is reframed as something other than a security threat even though some form of menace or conflict may still be present; *replacement*, which is when one issue is diminished in significance while being replaced by another; *rearticulation*, which occurs when an issue is recast as a non-security issue due to a resolution of the underlying conditions that warranted its initial securitization; and *silencing*, which occurs when an issue is depoliticized but also side-lines potentially insecure referents (ibid., p. 529).

It is in this regard that by actively reframing its disease eradication responsibilities using alternative language and concepts more akin to conventional public health, the WHO secretariat's actions potentially align most closely with desecuritization via rearticulation. Said another way, by intentionally extracting the health-as-security discourse from its communications with member states and replacing it with health-related technocratic language, the IO is seeking to fundamentally transform the debate surrounding how best to deal with the problem of infectious disease outbreaks. The solution offered to address this issue is to strengthen the disease surveillance and response technical capacity under the IHR (2005) which, while once associated as essential to global health security, has now been reframed as a procedural state-building initiative (see Cassels et al. 2014, WHO 2014b). These measures, as Hansen (2012, p. 543) has observed, thereby seek to extract the rearticulated issue (infectious diseases) out of the Schmittian 'friend-enemy' distinction that would otherwise necessitate emergency measures and re-insert it into a forum whereby political contestation and debate over how best to deal with the problem (e.g. economic investment) resumes.

It is here, however, that the WHO secretariat may yet also confront one of its most significant and potentially insurmountable challenges. More precisely, given that the IO's securitization of health issues has proven to be so effective – as evidenced by such developments as the massive increases in funding to strengthen global preparedness, member states' almost universal development of pandemic preparedness plans, the passage of new legislation designed to facilitate intergovernmental (and intrastate) cooperation to combat infectious disease, and efforts to enable greater access to medicines via the creation of new global health partnerships – serious questions can be raised whether in fact the correlations that have now been drawn between health and security can be persuasively 'un-made'. This is a challenge that is best encapsulated by Jeff Huysmans (2002), so much so that it has since become known as 'the Huysmans dilemma' (Wæver 2011).

In short, Huysmans' dilemma recognizes the difficulty associated with successfully desecuritizing an issue without simultaneously making reference to – and thereby further reinforcing – the original securitization. Put more simply, how do you convincingly argue that an issue is no longer a security issue when in uttering those very words you have drawn attention to its pre-existing status and identification as a security threat? At a more fundamental level, what this dilemma highlights is the problematic nature of 'un-making' a speech act once it has been uttered/performed/acted and has entered the social world. For the WHO, which willingly co-opted the efforts of a number of high-income countries in drawing the world's attention to the physical, economic, social, and political dangers arising from fast-moving acute health hazards such as infectious diseases and bioweapons, and which persuasively argued that such 'threats' warrant emergency measures to mitigate, the problem now becomes how to encourage governments (and the leaders, policy-makers, and general public contained within) to forget these initial associations and re-imagine these issues in an alternative light.

For the WHO secretariat the problem is further compounded by the fact that even if the IO was able to effectively engender this new understanding, the unpredictability of events like disease outbreaks or bioterrorist attacks, combined with their impact on human physical and mental well-being, inhibits the normalization of these incidents. The randomness and the existential and psychological impact automatically disrupts customary social patterns, which in turn necessitates the prioritization of response. The very nature of such events thus demands that they receive priority, and as Buzan et al. (1998, p. 24) have noted, an issue is usually designated as a security issue 'because it can be argued that this issue is more important than other issues and should take absolute priority'. The current outbreak of Ebola in West Africa thus serves as a manifest example, for in a world-first this latest outbreak has even warranted the deployment of thousands of military personnel to help contain the virus. As such, it is at least plausible that were the WHO now to successfully reframe its disease eradication mandate, locating it within a more traditional public health framework, the new frame will collapse as soon as another event materializes which exhibits the characteristics previously described as constituting a security threat. The risk to the WHO secretariat then transforms to one in which questions are raised about its performance, continued relevance, and whether the IO has been doing its job 'properly' or rather shirking its delegated duty.

For the moment, the above scenario remains purely hypothetical. What is clear, however, is that the WHO secretariat has currently set on a path to desecuritize its disease eradication delegation contract and return it to its former 'health-for-security' status, albeit while performing specific roles that have proved intrinsic to its health-as-security mandate. Presumably, these actions are being taken with the full knowledge and consent of the IO's leadership, and especially of the WHO director-general. As this book has demonstrated, the personal and professional experiences of those in leadership positions within the WHO have played a key role in shaping the direction of the organization – sometimes to the benefit and at times to the detriment of the IO's reputation. These findings are consistent with the work of others exploring IO independence, and as Oestreich (2012, p. 265) has observed, the importance of 'visionary leaders' at the helm of IOs cannot be overstated, principally because 'these are human institutions, run by people who are key variables in themselves'. Whether the WHO secretariat's latest decision to extricate itself from the health security discourse proves to be the latter or the former of these outcomes is yet to be revealed, but as the current director-general has no doubt shaped the policies and direction of the WHO, so too will the next person who assumes that role. It is also in this regard that securitization may return as a viable frame for the organization's activities at some point in the future – either in response to an internal change in policy focus, political pressure from member states, or in response to external events – but in the long run only time will tell.

It is also in this regard that the book has additionally attempted to reveal how rationalist and constructivist approaches can in fact be complementary. By using the PA theory model and examining the various shifts and turns in the WHO's approach to eradicating disease (and, importantly, the context in which they occurred), the book has been able to interrogate how a collective agent has attempted to shirk, slip, or address the stated collective preferences of its principals at various junctures. In blending this rationalist model with constructivism though, it has also revealed how both principals' and the agent's preferences have changed in response to events external to the IO as well as internal developments. Perhaps most importantly, it has also revealed how the WHO secretariat has collectively exercised discretion at times (Johnson and Urpelainen 2014), even when the opportunity arguably arose for the IO to engage in agency slack when confronted with considerable preference heterogeneity amongst its principals.

Ultimately, however, what this book has sought to highlight is the vitally important role that the WHO fulfils. Given that the IO was the first specialized UN agency ever to be created, it is somewhat surprising that the organization has attracted so little attention over the years. Of course, like any major bureaucracy, the WHO is subject to inefficiencies and failures. Opportunities have been squandered and resources have been wasted, much to the irritation of its member states – both the wealthy and the less so. The WHO and its secretariat are thus far from perfect. Equally though, the WHO secretariat – like many secretariats of intergovernmental organizations – faces a daunting task in attempting to meet the needs of almost 200 masters, all of which hold divergent views and differing opinions on what the organization should do and how it should do it. Programmes are commenced and staff are employed, but under the current funding arrangements where three quarters of the IO's budget is comprised of voluntary contributions, both can be terminated at a moment's notice if member states' priorities change.

The fact that the WHO has been able to accomplish so much within these arrangements should therefore perhaps be cautiously applauded.

It is also within this context that the WHO secretariat's forswearing of the global health security discourse is somewhat lamentable. Indeed, for all the criticisms and negative consequences that have been attributed to the securitization of a certain sub-set of health issues, it conceivably could still prove to be a very valuable political tool for improving the health outcomes of people all over the world due to the simple fact that security, like sex, sells. It should never be forgotten, for instance, that for decades wealthier countries willingly neglected a host of infectious diseases because they had been largely eliminated from within their respective territories. Globalization and the realization that these diseases are no longer geographically constrained, combined with the framing of these pathogens as 'threats', re-ignited the international community's attention and spurred considerable financial investment into strengthening disease surveillance and health systems around the world. That this investment had a distorting impact should not be overlooked, but as Hoffman (2010, p. 516) has optimistically noted, 'this situation may be improving over time. Certain redistributional consequences, for example, are likely to emerge as the health security interests of wealthier countries increasingly align with the social and economic goals of less developed countries'. Rather than discard the health-as-security discourse and disengage from diplomatic discussions that utilize this frame, therefore, perhaps the more appropriate, ethical course of action, as Hwenda et al. (2011, p. 21) have argued, is to ensure that low-income countries use such opportunities 'in order to advance their health security interests'. Fortunately, a forum already exists through which such arguments can be actively prosecuted – the WHA.

Moreover, as noted above, now that the connections have been drawn so successfully, it remains highly problematic for the IO to fully reverse course by discarding the health-as-security discourse without consequences ensuing. Instead, a far more productive use of both the IO's and member states' time would be to re-focus collective efforts on resolving the definitional problems surrounding the concept of global health security. It is clear, for instance, from WHA deliberations that even some of those member states that have previously railed against the IO's use of the phrase 'health security' in relation to the organization's work have periodically exploited the terminology for their own domestic and international objectives. From this it may be ascertained that the assumed preference heterogeneity over global health security may be more reflective of intermittent political posturing for domestic political gain rather than resolute, outright hostility, and as such, definitional consensus may in fact be attainable. The question thus becomes whether the political will to tackle this problem exists within the WHO secretariat, or whether it is far easier to move on to other issues.

In this book, the position explicitly adopted has been to support a narrow definition – one that embraces fast-moving, acute hazards to human health such as infectious diseases while excluding others. Such a narrow definition aligns with the WHO's founding raison d'être and delegation contract. It also parallels the PHEIC concept that has been articulated and enshrined within the revised IHR (2005), as well as the WHO's customary practice that has emerged since the turn of the century. Perhaps most compelling, however, is that a narrow definition of global health security that focuses on the control and elimination of infectious diseases coincides with the majority view of policy-makers and academics (Rushton 2011; see also DeLaet 2015, Stevenson and Moran 2015, Weir 2015 for examples). Alternative definitions, of course, have emerged at the margins and are likely to continue to do so (see Aldis 2008, McInnes 2015 for summaries). But as Rushton (2011, 2012) has articulated, there is the sense that we do already have a clear understanding of what the concept pertains to and that is, ultimately, the control (and wherever possible eradication) of infectious diseases.

Agreeing on a narrow definition does not preference either a state-centric or human security paradigm though, as Rushton (2011, pp. 787–793) suggests. Indeed, given the ongoing level of human suffering, morbidity, and mortality arising from infectious diseases as well as the potential for damage to national economies and social functioning, health security is arguably one instance where government and individual security interests fuse. It is conceivably for these reasons that even some of the staunchest detractors of the WHO's adoption of the concept have used health security for their own purposes, as outlined earlier. Therefore, rather than seeking to perpetuate an unhelpful debate as to which worldview of security should dominate, in this instance the international community would be better served by addressing the continuing technical capacity gaps that reside at the domestic and international levels and that preclude the WHO from fulfilling its mandate.

Technical and human resource capacity gaps linger as the international community's most pressing inhibitor for improving global health. These cavities also continue to thwart full compliance with the revised IHR (2005) (Davies et al. 2015). Disturbingly, these gaps were well known prior to the 2003 SARS outbreak and provided a powerful motivation for the WHO secretariat to issue travel advisories in an attempt to prevent the pathogen gaining a foothold in low-income countries, particularly Africa (Heymann 2005). Multiple resource-poor countries also went to considerable effort to stress during the IHR IGWG that in agreeing to the revised framework deemed so critical to ensuring global health, security was an expectation that the world's wealthier countries would assist their less wealthy counterparts develop the requisite core capacities in disease surveillance and outbreak response. Yet throughout the intervening years between the adoption of the revised IHR (2005) and the deadline for full compliance, the majority of high-income countries offered very little in the way of assistance. For a time it may have appeared that the lack of action was justifiable, especially in the wake of the global financial crisis that the 'threat' narrative was overblown. As the most recent outbreak of Ebola in West Africa has profoundly demonstrated again though, the level of physical, temporal, and cognitive interconnectedness that now permeates our world cannot be easily discarded, and the same measures that facilitate global trade also enable worldwide microbial dissemination. The perennial challenge for improving health systems to combat the spread of infectious diseases thus remains, and it behoves the international community to arrive at innovative solutions.

In this respect, one of the more interesting features of the current response to Ebola in West Africa has been the deployment of thousands of military personnel to help contain the outbreak. Military intervention in global health has been a topic of fierce debate over the years, with the overwhelming majority of commentators from non-governmental, public health, and even military disciplines arguing against such measures (Elbe 2006, Feldbaum et al. 2006, Bernard 2013). Some have even postulated that the comingling of health and security has resulted in a medicalization of security policy (Elbe 2010b). Despite this, however, military forces have a long-established interest in mitigating the spread of infectious diseases and considerable logistical and medical expertise that can substantially aid civilian efforts (Smith 1992, Owens et al. 2009, Kronmen et al. 2013). Encouraging greater civil-military cooperation in health security may provide an innovative and sustainable pathway to addressing capacity gaps in light of the financial constraints and the reduction in health-related ODA that have emerged in recent years, and yet the conventional position adopted by most health advocates and policy entrepreneurs decries such notions. If capacity gaps are to be addressed, however, pioneering measures are required and civil-military cooperation may offer one avenue of possibility.

Of course, capacity building will take years to accomplish. In the meantime it may be tempting for member states – given the self-acknowledged dysfunction of the WHO's latest efforts to prevent the spread of a highly lethal contagion in the form of Ebola – to move swiftly to impose yet further mechanisms of control on the IO to prevent further agency slack. Without addressing the budgetary issues though, any such moves would be short-sighted to say the least. Plainly there is need for further administrative and programmatic reform, but simply reducing the WHO's voluntary contributions and curtailing its staff is hardly the way to achieve this. Here the organization's proximal principals have the greatest responsibility to ensure that the reforms that are implemented will result in a leaner, more effective IO as opposed to applying measures that will cause additional dysfunction. The WHO is, ultimately, the sum of its parts and due to the limitations enshrined within its delegation contract, the IO's autonomy remains appropriately limited.

The fight against infectious diseases is far from over. Indeed aside from the periodic appearance of new zoonotic diseases that have successfully managed to cross the species barrier to infect humans (such as Ebola, SARS, and MERS-CoV), the emergence and progressive spread of AMR that the international community is presently witnessing reveals how limited modern medicine – for all our medical advances – really is at present. When viewed against the technological advances that are permitting humans to travel further and faster than ever before, the prospect of a disease-free future does not look particularly promising at the moment. The WHO's central mission and mandate have thus never been more important, and yet while the organization is in need of further reform to ensure greater efficiencies, equally the IO arguably needs the financial and political backing of its principals now more than ever. It is, after all, those governments and the people they represent that the WHO exists to serve.

Notes

Introduction

1   It is often assumed in PA theory that agents exhibit preference homogeneity by always seeking to maximize organizational autonomy and expansion of existing mandates and authority – see Weaver (2007) and Elsig (2010).
2   The use of the term 'proximal principals' is distinct from 'proximate principals' as described by Nielson and Tierney (2003) and Weaver (2007). More specifically, Nielson and Tierney (2003, p. 249) define it as 'the principal with the formal authority to hire, fire, or otherwise alter the agent's employment contract', whereas Weaver (2007, p. 498) uses it to differentiate between the 'most powerful member states' and other principals. The use of the term here, therefore, aligns more with Weaver's definition but is intended to signal how the IO views certain member states as more important to its mission than others.

1   The Legal Basis for the WHO's Global Health Security Mandate and Authority

1   The idea for a new universal health agency was first proposed in 1946 by the Chinese and Brazilian delegations attending the UN conference in San Francisco, but it took another two years before the requisite number of member states had signed and ratified the treaty to officially create the WHO.
2   The 1851 agreement was ratified by France and Sardinia, but in 1865 Sardinia withdrew, resulting in the regulations becoming defunct (see WHO, 1958, p. 7).
3   The Staff Regulations of the WHO were first adopted by the Fourth WHA in 1951 under resolution WHA4.51 and were subsequently amended by the 12th (1959), 55th (2002), and 62nd (2009) WHAs (see resolutions WHA12.33, WHA55.21, and WHA62.7).

2   The WHO's Classical Approach to Disease Eradication

1   The exception to this goal was the elimination of all forms of human malaria throughout Africa, which was deemed to be unattainable at the time due to the poor health infrastructure (see Fenner et al. 1988, pp. 381–382).
2   Several senior WHO officials had formerly trained as malariologists. They included, for example, Dr Candau, the WHO director-general; Dr Fred L. Soper, President of the PASB; and Dr Emilio Pampana, Member of the Secretariat of the Interim Commission of the WHO and later Secretary of the Expert Committee on Malaria (see Farid 1980, p. 12; Gramiccia and Beales 1988, p. 1345; Black 1986, pp. 117–121; and Cockburn 1961, p. 1051).

3 The WHO did adopt a second strategy in the MEP, focusing on the use of chloroquine-based anti-malarial drugs. Nevertheless, the central control strategy focused overwhelmingly on DDT residual spraying – see WHO 1960b, pp. 1–7.

4 The use of monetary rewards for the reporting of undetected smallpox cases became increasingly used as a method in the later years of the SEP, with rewards of up to US$1,000 eventually being offered (see Fenner et al. 1988, p. 538; Glynn and Glynn 2004, p. 209; and Joarder et al. 1980, p. 44). Other ingenious methods were also utilized by national campaigns; for example, one inspired innovation occurred in India, where infected beggars were temporarily housed and given food, clothing, and money. The effect also served to simultaneously isolate them and thereby prevent further transmission (see Glynn and Glynn 2004, pp. 211–212).

5 The Regional Director of the Americas had requested to re-allocate SEP funds to fighting malaria – see Fenner et al. 1988, p. 462. Thus, had the director-general permitted the re-allocation of regional funds, it is likely that it would have alienated the Americas branch of the WHO; given that the United States was one of the SEP's largest donors, this would have been an undesirable outcome.

6 A select number of instances were recorded where local authorities attempted to conceal the presence of smallpox epidemics from national authorities and WHO personnel (see, for example, Basu et al. 1979, pp. 294–296; see also Glynn and Glynn 2004, pp. 203, 213). A further instance also occurred in Somalia in September 1976, resulting in WHO personnel being prevented from undertaking vital fieldwork in an attempt to contain an epidemic (see Fenner et al. 1988, p. 536 and Glynn and Glynn 2004, p. 223).

7 Variations on this slogan were also adopted by national campaigns to distinguish the intensified programme. For example, India's intensified campaign became referred to as 'Operation Smallpox Zero' (see Basu et al. 1979, pp. 32–34).

3 Securitization and SARS: A New Framing?

1 Although the Chinese government objected to resolution WHA54.14, as mentioned below, it is important to note that their criticism did not relate to the definition of global health security as articulated by the WHO secretariat.

2 Only one member state, the People's Republic of China, was identified as advocating that the conventional system of disease notification should be maintained – see WHO 2001b.

4 New Powers for a New Age? Revising and Updating the IHR

1 The five clinical syndromes included acute haemorrhagic fever syndrome, acute respiratory syndrome, acute diarrhoeal syndrome, acute neurological syndrome, and acute jaundice syndrome.

2 Although three IGWG meetings were held, on 1–12 November 2004; 21–26 February 2005; and in May 2005, officially the IGWG convened in only two sessions (November 2004 and February/May 2005), with the second session being suspended for a period of approximately three months before reconvening and finalizing the negotiations.

3 Under Article 18 of the revised IHR (2005), the WHO secretariat is authorized to issue recommendations to member states to 'review travel history in affected areas' with respect to persons, but again, a strict interpretation of this article would not permit the secretariat to publicly issue travel advisories – only member states.

5 Pandemic Influenza: 'The Most Feared Security Threat'

1 David L. Heymann was only appointed as Assistant Director-General for the Health Security and Environment Cluster following Dr Margaret Chan's appointment as WHO director-general, which followed Dr Jong-wook Lee's untimely death on 22 May 2006.

6 Global Health Security and Its Discontents

1 For example, the authors claim that the director-general securitized the 2009 H1N1 influenza virus by declaring a PHEIC and announcing a pandemic (p. 9), although these claims ignore the revised IHR (2005) requirements under Annex 2 that a novel influenza virus with human-to-human transmission qualifies as a PHEIC – a factor that, critically, was negotiated and approved by the IO's member states throughout the IHR IGWG and later endorsed by the 58th WHA. It also overlooks the role of the IHR Emergency Committee in the director-general's ability to declare a PHEIC, and indeed Dr Chan did not elevate the alert level to phase 6 (full pandemic) until the IHR Emergency Committee recommended that the alert level be raised. Further, the authors' claims that additional oversight mechanisms are warranted to curb the risk of the WHO secretariat exceeding its authority via the invocation of emergency powers overlooks the existing role of the EB, the IO's internal legal counsel, as well as the IHR Emergency Committee.

2 While no mention of 'global health security' was included in the EB resolution pertaining to the IHR (*EB122.R3 Implementation of the International Health Regulations [2005]*), intriguingly the phrase did appear in resolution *EB122.R4 Climate change and health* – see WHO EB (2008b).

3 It is important to note that the WHO's medium-term strategic plan was originally released in 2008, but then revised and re-released in 2009. Although the WHO's content of both versions of these plans remains largely the same, for the purposes of this book the revised strategic plan has been used for analysis.

4 For example, the WHO Regional Office for Africa assisted countries that included Malawi, Lesotho, Swaziland, and Mauritius to develop a range of country cooperation strategies – see WHO AFRO (2009a, 2009b, 2009c, 2009d). See also WHO (2008d).

5   The only explicit reference to 'global health security' in all of the 66th WHA secretariat's reports to member states can be found in relation to the report on mass gatherings; importantly, member states were only invited to consider the report and no resolution or further action was required – see WHO (2012h).

6   As noted in an information document, although the final report was not submitted to the EB until January 2011, a number of consultations were held with member states throughout 2010 on the preliminary findings of the organization-wide review – see WHO EB (2010b).

7   It would be inaccurate to suggest that the WHO secretariat was forced to abandon its use of the phrase 'global health security', as the evidence does not support this. For while there was a small but vocal group of protagonists that objected to the IO's use of this discourse, there is no evidence to indicate a widespread movement. As such, the only conclusion that can be drawn is that the WHO willingly discarded the concept.

8   For example, new interim case definitions were released by the WHO on 25 September 2012, 29 September 2012, 16 January 2013, 19 February 2013, and 3 July 2013.

9   Ebola did not appear in Spain until early October 2014.

10 According to Cheng (2014), serious concerns about the WHO's lack of attentiveness were identified by MSF in April 2014, resulting in the WHO criticizing MSF for politicizing the outbreak and for a breakdown of trust.

11 According to Cheng (2014), serious concerns about the WHO's response to the Ebola outbreak were raised by MSF in April 2014.

Bibliography

Abraham T (2005) *Twenty-First Century Plague: The Story of SARS*. Baltimore: Johns Hopkins University Press.

Abraham T (2011) The Chronicle of a Disease Foretold: Pandemic H1N1 and the Construction of a Global Health Security Threat. *Political Studies*, 59(4): 797–812.

Aginam O and Rupiya M (eds) (2012) *HIV/AIDS and the Security Sector in Africa* Tokyo: United Nations University Press.

Aldis W (2008) Health Security as a Public Health Concept: A Critical Analysis. *Health Policy and Planning*, 23: 369–75.

Alvarez JE (2005) *International Organizations as Law-makers*. Oxford: Oxford University Press.

Amorim C, Douste-Blazy P, Wirayuda H, Støre JG, Gadio CT, Dlamini-Zuma N and Pibulsonggram N (2007) Oslo Ministerial Declaration-Global Health: A Pressing Foreign Policy Issue of Our Time. *The Lancet*, 369(9570): 1373–8.

Anonymous (2005) Interview with Senior WHO Official, 14 November 2005. Geneva: Switzerland.

Aradau C (2004) Security and the Democratic Scene: Desecuritization and Emancipation. *Journal of International Relations and Development*, 7(4): 388–413.

Ashraf H (2003) China Finally Throws Full Weight Behind Efforts to Contain SARS. *The Lancet*, 361(9367): 1439.

Ashworth LM (1999) *Creating International Studies: Angell, Mitrany and the Liberal Tradition*. Aldershot: Ashgate.

Ashworth LM (2005) David Mitrany and South-East Europe: The Balkan Key to World Peace. *The Historical Review*, 2: 203–24.

Asian Development Bank (2003) *Outlook 2003 Update: Trends, Analysis, Projections*. Manila: Asian Development Bank.

Baker M and Fidler D (2006) Global Public Health Surveillance under New International Health Regulations. *Emerging Infectious Diseases*, 12(7): 1058–65.

Bale HE (2002) Patents, Patients and Developing Countries: Access, Innovation and the Political Dimensions of Trade Policy. In Granville B (ed) *The Economics of Essential Medicines*. London: Royal Institute of International Affairs: 100–10.

Balzacq T (2011) A Theory of Securitization: Origins, Core Assumptions, and Variants. In Balzacq T (ed) *Securitization Theory: How Security Problems Emerge and Resolve*. Oxon: Routledge: 1–30.

Banerjee A (2010) Tracking of Global Funding for the Prevention and Control of Non-communicable Diseases. *Bulletin of the World Health Organization*, 90(7): 479.

Barberis DS (2003) In Search of an Object: Organicist Sociology and the Reality of Society in *fin-de-siècle* France. *History of the Human Sciences*, 16(3): 51–72.

Barnett M and Finnemore M (1999) The Politics, Power, and Pathologies of International Organizations. *International Organization*, 53(4): 699–732.

Barnett M and Finnemore M (2004) *Rules for the World: International Organizations in Global Politics.* London: Cornell University Press.

Basu R, Jezek Z and Ward N (1979) *The Eradication of Smallpox in India.* WHO Series History of International Public Health No. 2. India: World Health Organization.

Beales P and Gilles H (2002) Rationale and Technique of Malaria Control. In Warrell D and Gilles H (eds) *Essential Malariology.* 4th edition. London: Arnold: 107–90.

Beigbeder Y (1987) *Management Problems in United Nations Organizations: Reform or Decline?* London: Frances Pinter.

Beigbeder Y (1998) *The World Health Organization.* The Hague: Martinus Nijhoff.

Bell D and WHO Working Group on Prevention of International and Community Transmission of SARS (2004) Public Health Interventions and SARS Spread, 2003. *Emerging Infectious Diseases,* 10(11): 1900–6.

Benatar SR (2001) Respiratory Health in a Globalizing World. *American Journal of Respiratory and Critical Care Medicine,* 163(5): 1064–7.

Benford RD and Snow DA (2000) Framing Processes and Social Movements: An Overview and Assessment. *Annual Review of Sociology,* 26(4): 611–39.

Bernard K (2013) Health and National Security: A Contemporary Collision of Cultures. *Biosecurity and Bioterrorism,* 11(2): 157–62.

Bhopal R (2002) *Concepts of Epidemiology: An Integrated Introduction to the Ideas, Theories, Principles and Methods of Epidemiology.* Oxford: Oxford University Press.

Black M (1986) *The Children and the United Nations: The Story of Unicef.* Sydney: UNICEF.

Bøås M and McNeill D (2004) Power and Ideas in Multilateral Institutions: Towards an Interpretative Framework. In Bøås M and McNeill D (eds) *Global Institutions & Development: Framing the World?* London: Routledge: 1–12.

Boseley S (2012) Polio Eradication Effort Stumbles Again after Murders of Five Women in Pakistan. *The Guardian.co.uk,* 18 December 2012. Accessed 20 January 2013. http://www.guardian.co.uk/world/2012/dec/18/polio-eradication-effort-stumbles-again

Brandt AM and Gardner M (2000) Antagonism and Accommodation: Interpreting the Relationship Between Public Health and Medicine in the United States During the 20th Century. *American Journal of Public Health,* 90(5): 707–15.

Brès P (1986) *Public Health Action in Emergencies Caused by Epidemics: A Practical Guide.* Geneva: World Health Organization.

Bresalier M (2011) Fighting Flu: Military Pathology, Vaccines, and the Conflicted Identity of the 1918–19 Pandemic in Britain. *Journal of History of Medicine and Allied Sciences,* 68(1): 87–128.

Briggs A (1961) Cholera and Society in the Nineteenth Century. *Past and Present,* 19(1): 76–96.

Brookes T (2005) *Behind the Mask: How the World Survived SARS. The First Epidemic of the Twenty-First Century.* Washington, DC: American Public Health Association.

Brown D (2009) System Set Up After SARS Epidemic Was Slow to Alert Global Authorities. *The Washington Post,* 30 April 2009. Accessed 27 July 2014. http://www.washingtonpost.com/wp-dyn/content/article/2009/04/29/AR2009042904911.html

Bruce-Chwatt LJ (1998) History of Malaria from Prehistory to Eradication. In Wernsdorfer W and McGregor I (eds) *Malaria: Principles and Practice of Malariology. Volume 1.* Edinburgh: Churchill Livingstone: 1–59.

Brundtland GH (2006) Personal Email Correspondence with Author, 13 April 2006. London.

Burci GL and Vignes C (2004) *World Health Organization.* The Hague: Kluwer.

Buzan B, Wæver O and de Wilde J (1998) *Security: A New Framework for Analysis.* London: Lynne Rienner.

Calain P (2007) Exploring the International Arena of Global Public Health Surveillance. *Health Policy and Planning,* 22(1): 2–12.

Calder R (1958) *Ten Steps Forward: World Health 1948–1958.* Geneva: World Health Organization.

Canagarajah S (1996) "Nondiscursive" Requirements in Academic Publishing, Material Resources of Periphery Scholars, and the Politics of Knowledge Production. *Written Communication,* 13(4): 435–72.

Carrin GJ (2006) Rousseau's "Social Contract": Contracting Ahead of Its Time? *Bulletin of the World Health Organization,* 84(11): 917–18.

Carter I (1982) Communication and Disease. *Proceedings of the Royal Society of Edinburgh. Section B. Biological Sciences,* 82: 101–15.

Cassels A, Smith I and Burci GL (2014) Reforming the WHO: The Art of the Possible. *Public Health,* 128(2): 202–4.

Cassese A (2005) *International Law.* 2nd edition. Oxford: Oxford University Press.

Castillo-Salgado C (2010) Trends and Directions of Global Public Health Surveillance. *Epidemiologic Reviews,* 32(1): 93–109. doi:10.1093/epirev/mxq008.

Cegielski JP, Chin DP, Espinal MA, Frieden TR, Cruz RR, Talbot EA, Weil DE, Zaleskis R and Raviglione MC (2002) The Global Tuberculosis Situation: Progress and Problems in the 20th Century, Prospects for the 21st Century. *Infectious Disease Clinics of North America,* 16(1): 1–58.

Chang WC (2002) The Meaning and Goals of Equity in Health. *Journal of Epidemiology and Community Health,* 56: 488–91.

Chen C, Chien Y and Yang H (2003) Epidemiology and Control of Severe Acute Respiratory Syndrome (SARS) Outbreak in Taiwan. In Koh T, Plant A and Lee E (eds) *The New Global Threat: Severe Acute Respiratory Syndrome and Its Impacts.* Singapore: World Scientific: 301–16.

Cheng M (2014) UN: We Botched Response to the Ebola Outbreak. Associated Press, 17 October 2014. Accessed 8 November 2014. http://hosted2.ap.org/APDEFAULT/3d281c11a96b4ad082fe88aa0db04305/Article_2014-10-17-EU-MED--WHO%20Ebola%20Mistakes/id-d2ad1e1bada6470388893ac1c4111137

Chorev N (2012) *The World Health Organization between North and South.* Ithaca: Cornell University Press.

Cochi SL, De Quadros CA, Dittmann S, Foster SO, Galvez Tan JZ, Grant FC, Olive JM, Pigman HA, Taylor CE and Wang K (1998) Group Report: What Are the Societal and Political Criteria for Disease Eradication. In Dowdle WR and Hopkins DR (eds) *The Eradication of Infectious Diseases.* Chichester: John Wiley & Sons: 157–75.

Cockburn A (1961) Eradication of Infectious Diseases. *Science,* 133(3458): 1050–8.

Cocksedge S (2009) Personal Email Correspondence with Author, 18 June 2009. London.

Cohen E (2009) When a Pandemic isn't a Pandemic. *CNN*, 4 May 2009. Accessed 27 July 2014. http://edition.cnn.com/2009/HEALTH/05/04/swine.flu.pandemic/index.html

Cohen HW, Gould RM and Sidel VW (2004) The Pitfalls of Bioterrorism Preparedness: The Anthrax and Smallpox Experiences. *American Journal of Public Health*, 94(10): 1667–71.

Cohen M, Naik G and Pottinger M (2003) Spreading the Word: Inside WHO as It Mobilized for War on SARS. *The Wall Street Journal*, 2 May 2003, A1.

Collier S and Lakoff A (2008) The Problem of Securing Health. In Lakoff A and Collier S (eds) *Biosecurity Interventions: Global Health and Security in Question.* New York: Colombia University Press: 7–32.

Cortell A and Peterson S (2006) Dutiful Agents, Rogue Actors, or Both? Staffing, Voting Rules, and Slack in the WHO and WTO. In Hawkins D, Lake D, Nielson D and Tierney M (eds) *Delegation and Agency in International Organizations.* Cambridge: Cambridge University Press: 255–80.

Cox R and Jacobsen HK (1973) *The Anatomy of Influence.* Cambridge: Cambridge University Press.

Crampton T (2003) W.H.O. Criticizes China Over Handling of Mystery Disease. *The New York Times*, 7 April 2003. Accessed 26 July 2014. http://www.nytimes.com/2003/04/07/international/asia/07CND-HONG.html

Curley M and Herington J (2011) The Securitization of Avian Influenza: International Discourses and Domestic Politics in Asia. *Review of International Studies*, 37(1): 141–66.

Davenport F (1979) The Search for the Ideal Influenza Vaccine. *Postgraduate Medical Journal*, 55(640): 78–86.

Davies S (2008) Securitizing Infectious Diseases. *International Affairs*, 84(2): 295–313.

Davies S (2010) *Global Politics of Health.* Cambridge: Polity.

Davies S (2012) Duty in the Time of Epidemics: What China and Zimbabwe Teach Us. *Australian Journal of International Affairs*, 66(4): 413–30.

Davies S (2015) Internet surveillance and disease outbreaks. In Rushton S and Youde J (eds) *Routledge Handbook of Global Health Security.* Abingdon: Routledge: 226–38.

Davies S, Kamradt-Scott A and Rushton S (2015) *Disease Diplomacy: International Norms and Global Health Security.* Baltimore: Johns Hopkins University Press.

Davis JW (2012) A Critical View of Global Governance. *Swiss Political Science Review*, 18: 272–86.

DeLaet D (2015) Whose Interests is the Securitization of Health Serving? In Rushton S and Youde J (eds) *Routledge Handbook of Global Health Security.* Abingdon: Routledge: 339–48.

Delon PJ (1975) *The International Health Regulations: A Practical Guide.* Geneva: World Health Organization.

Doshi P (2011) The Elusive Definition of Pandemic Influenza. *Bulletin of the World Health Organization*, 89(7): 532–8.

Doull JA (1948) The First World Health Assembly. *Public Health Reports*, 63(43): 1379–410.

Dowdle WR (1999) Influenza A Virus Recycling Revisited. *Bulletin of the World Health Organization*, 77(10): 820–8.

Duffin J and Sweetman A (eds) (2006) *SARS in Context: Memory, History, Policy.* Montreal: McGill-Queen's University Press.

Dutt S (1995) *The Politicization of the United Nations Specialized Agencies: A Case Study of UNESCO*. Lampeter: Mellen University Press.

Edelman S (1963) International Travel and Our National Quarantine System. *Temple Law Quarterly*, 37: 28–40.

Elbe S (2003) *Strategic Implications of HIV/AIDS*. Adephi Paper 357. Oxford: International Institute for Strategic Studies.

Elbe S (2006) Should HIV/AIDS be Securitized? The Ethical Dilemmas of Linking HIV/AIDS and Security. *International Studies Quarterly*, 50(1): 119–44.

Elbe S (2009) *Virus Alert: Security, Governmentality, and the AIDS Pandemic*. Columbia: Columbia University Press.

Elbe S (2010a) Haggling Over Viruses: The Downside Risks of Securitizing Infectious Disease. *Health Policy and Planning*, 25(6): 476–85.

Elbe S (2010b) *Security and Global Health*. Cambridge: Polity.

Elbe S (2011) Pandemics on the Radar Screen: Health Security, Infectious Disease and the Medicalisation of Insecurity. *Political Studies*, 59(4): 848–66.

Elbe S, Roemer-Mahler A and Long C (2014) Securing Circulation Pharmaceutically: Antiviral Stockpiling and Pandemic Preparedness in the European Union. *Security Dialogue*, Published online 23 May 2014, doi:10.1177/0967010614530072.

Elgie R (2002) The Politics of the European Central Bank: Principal-Agent Theory and the Democratic Deficit. *Journal of European Public Policy*, 9: 186–200.

Elling R (1981) The Capitalist-World System and International Health. *International Journal of Health Services*, 11(1): 21–51.

Elsig M (2010) Principal-Agent Theory and the World Trade Organization: Complex Agency and 'Missing Delegation'. *European Journal of International Relations*, 17(3): 495–517.

Enemark C (2009) Is Pandemic Flu a Security Threat?. *Survival*, 51(1): 191–214.

European Commission (2010) Avian Influenza as a Global Challenge. Archived Website. Accessed 5 June 2014. http://ec.europa.eu/world/avian_influenza/

FAO and OIE (2007) *The Global Strategy for Prevention and Control of H5N1 Highly Pathogenic Avian Influenza*. Geneva: Food and Agriculture Organization. Accessed 5 June 2014. http://www.fao.org/docs/eims/upload/210745/glob_strat_hpai_apr07_en.pdf

Farid MA (1980) The Malaria Program – From Euphoria to Anarchy. *World Health Forum*, 1(1&2): 8–33.

Fauci AS (2003) Infectious Diseases: Considerations for the 21st Century. *CID*, 32(March): 675–85.

Fee E and Brown T (2002) 100 Years of the Pan American Health Organization. *American Journal of Public Health*, 92(12): 1888–9.

Fee E and Parry M (2008) Jonathan Mann, HIV/AIDS, and Human Rights. *Journal of Public Health Policy*, 29(1): 54–71.

Feldbaum H, Patel P, Sondorp E and Lee K (2006) Global Health and National Security: The Need for Critical Engagement. *Medicine, Conflict and Survival*, 22(3): 192–8.

Fenner F, Henderson DA, Arita I, Jezek Z and Ladnyi ID (1988) *Smallpox and Its Eradication*. Geneva: World Health Organization.

Fidler DP (1996) Globalization, International Law, and Emerging Infectious Diseases. *Emerging Infectious Diseases*, 2(2): 77–84.

Fidler DP (1999) *International Law and Infectious Diseases*. Oxford: Clarendon.

Fidler DP (2004) *SARS, Governance and the Globalization of Disease*. London: Palgrave Macmillan.

Fidler DP (2005) From International Sanitary Conventions to Global Health Security: The New International Health Regulations. *Chinese Journal of International Law*, 4(2): 325–92.

Fidler DP (2014) Ebola and Global Health Governance: Time for the Reckoning. Royal Institute of International Affairs (Chatham House) Expert Comment. Accessed 8 November 2014. http://www.chathamhouse.org/expert/comment/15811

Fidler DP and Gostin L (2008) *Biosecurity in the Global Age: Biological Weapons, Public Health, and the Rule of Law*. Stanford: Stanford University Press.

Fink S (2014a) Cuts at W.H.O. Hurt Response to Ebola Crisis. *The New York Times*, 3 September 2014. Accessed 8 November 2014. http://www.nytimes.com/2014/09/04/world/africa/cuts-at-who-hurt-response-to-ebola-crisis.html?_r=0

Fink S (2014b) W.H.O. Leader Describes the Agency's Ebola Operations. *The New York Times*, 4 September 2014. Accessed 10 November 2014. http://www.nytimes.com/2014/09/04/world/africa/who-leader-describes-the-agencys-ebola-operations.html?_r=0

Fischer F (2003) *Reframing Public Policy: Discursive Politics and Deliberative Practices*. Oxford: Oxford University Press.

Fischer F and Katz R (2013) Moving Forward to 2014: Global IHR (2005) Implementation. *Biosecurity and Bioterrorism*, 11(2): 153–6.

Flahault A, Dias-Ferrao V, Chaberty P, Esteves K, Valleron AJ and Lavanchy D (1998) FluNet as a Tool for Global Monitoring of Influenza on the Web. *JAMA*, 280(15): 1330–2.

Fleck F (2004) West Africa Polio Campaign Boycotted by Nigerian States. *BMJ*, 328(7438): 485.

Francis T (1947) A Consideration of Vaccination against Influenza. *The Milbank Memorial Fund Quarterly*, 25(1): 5–20.

Gagnon M and Labonté R (2013) Understanding How and Why Health is Integrated into Foreign Policy – A Case Study of Health is Global, a UK Government Strategy 2008–13. *Globalization and Health*, 9(24): 1–19.

Gale J and Lauerman J (2014) How the World's Top Health Body Allowed Ebola to Spiral Out of Control. *Bloomberg.com*, 18 October 2014. Accessed 8 November 2014. http://www.bloomberg.com/news/2014-10-16/who-response-to-ebola-outbreak-foundered-on-bureaucracy.html

Gautier L, Harmer A, Tediosi F and Missoni E (2014) Reforming the World Health Organization: What Influence Do the BRICS Wield? *Contemporary Politics*, 20(2): 163–81.

Ghendon Y (1991) Influenza Surveillance. *Bulletin of the World Health Organization*, 69(5): 509–15.

Girard M, Tam J, Assossou O and Kieny M (2010) The 2009 A (H1N1) Influenza Virus Pandemic: A Review. *Vaccine*, 28(31): 4895–902.

Glynn I and Glynn J (2004) *The Life and Death of Smallpox*. London: Profile.

Godlee F (1994) The World Health Organization: WHO in Crisis. *BMJ*, 309(6966): 1424–8.

Godlee F (2010) Conflicts of Interest and Pandemic Flu. *BMJ*, 340: c2947.

Godlee F (2014) Phone Interview with Author, 26 September 2014. Launceston: Australia.

Goodman NM (1952) *International Health Organizations and Their Work*. Philadephia: Blakiston.

Gordenker L (2005) *The UN Secretary-General and Secretariat.* Oxon: Routledge.

Gostin L (2009) Influenza A (H1N1) and Pandemic Preparedness Under the Rule of International Law. *JAMA*, 301(22): 2376–8.

Gostin L and Phelan A (2014) The Global Health Security Agenda in an Age of Biosecurity. *JAMA*, 312(1): 27–8.

Global Polio Eradication Initiative (2013) History. Accessed 10 August 2013. http://www.polioeradication.org/Aboutus/History.aspx

Graham ER (2014) International Organizations as Collective Agents: Fragmentation and the Limits of Principal Control at the World Health Organization. *European Journal of International Relations*, 20(2): 366–90.

Gramiccia G and Beales PF (1988) The Recent History of Malaria Control and Eradication. In Wernsdorfer WH and McGregor I (eds) *Malaria: Principles and Practice of Malariology. Volume 2.* Edinburgh: Churchill Livingstone: 1335–78.

Green J and Colgan J (2012) Protecting Sovereignty, Protecting the Planet: State Delegation to International Organizations and Private Actors in Environmental Politics. *Governance*, doi:10.1111/j.1468-0491.2012.01607.x.

Greenberg DS (2002) War, Bioterrorism and the Political Landscape. *The Lancet*, 358(9299): 2137.

Grein T, Kamara K, Rodier G, Plant A, Bovier P, Ryan M, Ohyama T and Heymann DL (2000) Rumours of Disease in the Global Village: Outbreak Verification. *Emerging Infectious Diseases*, 6(2): 97–102.

Gupte MD, Ramachandran V and Mutatkar RT (2001) Epidemiological Profile in India: Historical and Contemporary Perspectives. *Journal of Biosciences*, 26 (4 Supp): 437–64.

Gutteridge F (1963) The World Health Organization: Its Scope and Achievements. *Temple Law Quarterly*, 37: 1–14.

Haas EB (1956) Regionalism, Functionalism, and Universal International Organization. *World Politics*, 8: 238–63.

Haas EB (1990) *When Knowledge is Power: Three Models of Change in International Organizations.* California: University of California Press.

Hale T and Held D (2012) Gridlock and Innovation in Global Governance: The Partial Transnational Solution. *Global Policy*, 3(2): 169–81.

Hampton BC (1925) International Health Organizations. *Public Health Reports (1896–1970)*, 40(34): 1719–93.

Hanrieder T and Kreuder-Sonnen C (2014) WHO Decides on the Exception? Securitization and Emergency Governance in Global Health. *Security Dialogue*, Published online 10 June 2014. doi:10.1177/0967010614535833.

Hansen L (2011) The Politics of Securitization and the Muhammad Cartoon Crisis: A Post-structuralist Perspective. *Security Dialogue*, 42(4–5): 357–69.

Hansen L (2012) Reconstructing Desecuritization: The Normative-Political in the Copenhagen School and Directions for How to Apply It. *Review of International Studies*, 38(3): 525–46.

Hardiman M (2003) The Revised International Health Regulations: A Framework for Global Health Security. *International Journal of Antimicrobial Agents*, 21(2): 207–11.

Harman S (2012) *Global Health Governance.* London: Routledge.

Harman S and Lisk F (eds) (2009) *Governance of HIV/AIDS: Making Participation and Accountability Count.* London: Routledge.

Hawkins D, Lake D, Nielson D and Tierney M (2006) Delegation under Anarchy: States, International Organizations, and Principal-Agent Theory. In Hawkins D, Lake D, Nielson D and Tierney M (eds) *Delegation and Agency in International Organizations*. Cambridge: Cambridge University Press: 3–38.

Hein W, Bartsch S and Kohlmorgen L (eds) (2007) *Global Health Governance and the Fight Against HIV/AIDS*. London: Palgrave Macmillan.

Henderson DA (1977) Smallpox Eradication. *Proceedings of the Royal Society of London*, 199(1134): 83–97.

Henderson DA (1987a) Smallpox Eradication: A WHO Success Story. *World Health Forum*, 8: 283–92.

Henderson DA (1987b) Principles and Lessons from the Smallpox Eradication Program. *Bulletin of the World Health Organization*, 65(4): 535–46.

Heymann D (2002) The Microbial Threat in Fragile Times: Balancing Known and Unknown Risks. *Bulletin of the World Health Organization*, 80(3): 179.

Heymann D (2003) Evolving Infectious Disease Threats to National and Global Security. In Chen L, Leaning J and Narasimhan V (eds) *Global Health Challenges for Human Security*. Cambridge: Harvard University Press: 105-23.

Heymann D (2004) The International Response to the Outbreak of SARS in 2003. *Philosophical Transactions of the Royal Society B*, 359(1447): 1127–9.

Heymann D (2005) Personal Interview with Author, 15 November 2005. Geneva: World Health Organization.

Heymann D (2009) Personal Interview with Author, 10 June 2009. London.

Heymann D and Aylward R (2004) Eradicating Polio. *New England Journal of Medicine*, 351(13): 1275–7.

Heymann D and Rodier G (1998) Global Surveillance of Communicable Diseases. *Emerging Infectious Diseases*, 4(3): 362–5.

Heymann D and Rodier G (2004a) SARS: A Global Response to an International Threat. *Brown Journal of World Affairs*, 10(2): 185–97.

Heymann D and Rodier G (2004b) Global Surveillance, National Surveillance, and SARS. *Emerging Infectious Diseases*, 10(2): 173–5.

Hodge J (2010) Global Legal Triage in Response to the 2009 H1N2 Outbreak. *Minnesota Journal of Law*, 11(2): 599–628.

Hoffman SJ (2010) The Evolution, Etiology and Eventualities of the Global Health Security Regime. *Health Policy and Planning*, 25(6): 510–22.

Holbrooke R and Garrett L (2008) 'Sovereignty' That Risks Global Health. *The Washington Post*, 10 August. Accessed 18 July 2014. http://www.washington-post.com/wp-dyn/content/article/2008/08/08/AR2008080802919.html

Hopkins JW (1989) *The Eradication of Smallpox: Organizational Learning and Innovation in International Health*. Colorado: Westview Press.

Horton R (2002) WHO Leadership: A Swift Start But with Few Clear Objectives. *The Lancet*, 360(9336): 812–13.

Howard-Jones N (1978) *International Public Health between the Two World Wars – The Organizational Problems*. Geneva: World Health Organization.

Huang Y (2011) The Sick Man of Asia: China's Health Crisis. *Foreign Affairs*, 90(6): 119–36.

Hughes JM (1998) Addressing Emerging Infectious Disease Threats – Accomplishments and Future Plans. *Emerging Infectious Diseases*, 4(3): 360–1.

Humphreys M (1996) Kicking a Dying Dog: DDT and the Demise of Malaria in the American South, 1942–1950. *Isis*, 87: 1–17.

Hussain M (2014) MSF Calls for Military Medics to Help Tackle West Africa Ebola. *Reuters Africa*, 2 September 2014. Accessed 8 November 2014. http://af.reuters.com/article/topNews/idAFKBN0GX1QP20140902

Huysmans J (2002) Defining Social Constructivism in Security Studies: The Normative Dilemma of Writing Security. *Alternatives*, 27(1): 41–64.

Hwenda L, Mahlathi P and Maphanga T (2011) Why African Countries Need to Participate in Global Health Security Discourse. *Global Health Governance*, 4(2): 1–24.

IHME (2012) *Financing Global Health 2012: The End of the Golden Age?* Seattle: Institute for Health Metrics and Evaluation.

IMCAPI (2008) The Sixth International Ministerial Conference on Avian and Pandemic Influenza, Sharm El-Sheikh, Egypt, 25–26 October 2008. Cairo: Government of Egypt. Accessed 5 June 2014. http://www.undg.org/docs/9517/GoE-final-SeS-statement.pdf

IMF (2006) *The Global Economic and Financial Impact of an Avian Flu Pandemic and the Role of the IMF*. Washington, DC: International Monetary Fund. Accessed 5 June 2014. http://www.imf.org/external/pubs/ft/afp/2006/eng/022806.pdf

Ingram A (2005) The New Geopolitics of Disease: Between Global Health and Global Security. *Geopolitics*, 10(3): 522–45.

Ingram A (2011) The Pentagon's HIV/AIDS Programmes: Governmentality, Political Economy, Security. *Geopolitics*, 16(3): 655–74.

Jensen K and Hogan R (1958) Laboratory Diagnosis of Asian Influenza. *Public Health Reports (1896–1970)*, 73(2): 140–4.

Jin J and Karackattu JT (2011) Infectious Diseases and Securitization: WHO's Dilemma. *Biosecurity and Bioterrorism*, 9(2): 181–7.

Joarder AK, Tarantola D and Tulloch J (1980) *The Eradication of Smallpox from Bangladesh*. WHO Regional Series Publications South-East Asia Series No. 8. New Delhi: WHO South-East Asia Regional Office.

Johnson T and Urpelainen J (2014) International Bureaucrats and the Formation of Intergovernmental Organizations: Institutional Design Discretion Sweetens the Pot. *International Organization*, 68(1): 177–209.

Kaiser R, Coulombier D, Baldari M, Morgan D and Paquet C (2006) What is Epidemic Intelligence, and How is It Being Improved in Europe? *Eurosurveillance*, 11(5): pii–2892. Accessed 26 July 2014. http://www.eurosurveillance.org/ViewArticle.aspx?ArticleId=2892

Kamradt-Scott A (2010) The WHO Secretariat, Norm Entrepreneurship, and Global Disease Outbreak Control. *Journal of International Organizations Studies*, 1(1): 72–89.

Kamradt-Scott A (2012) Changing Perceptions of Pandemic Influenza and Public Health Responses. *American Journal of Public Health*, 102(1): 90–8.

Kamradt-Scott A (2013) The Politics of Medicine and the Global Governance of Pandemic Influenza. *International Journal of Health Services*, 43(1): 105–21.

Kamradt-Scott A, Lee K and Xu J (2012) The International Health Regulations (2005): Asia's Contribution to a Global Health Governance Framework. In Lee K, Pang T and Tan Y (eds) *Asia's Role in Governing Global Health*. London: Routledge: 83-98.

Kamradt-Scott A and McInnes C (2012) The Securitization of Pandemic Influenza: Framing, Security and Public Policy. *Global Public Health*, 7(Supp 2): S95–110.

Karadesh J (2009) Wild Boars Killed in Iraq Over Swine Flu Fears. *CNN.com*, 3 May 2009. Accessed 27 July 2014. http://edition.cnn.com/2009/WORLD/meast/05/03/iraq.boars/

Kassim H and Menon A (2003) The Principal-Agent Approach and the Study of the European Union: Promise Unfulfilled? *Journal of European Public Policy*, 10(1): 121–39.

Katz R and Fischer J (2010) The Revised International Health Regulations: A Framework for Global Pandemic Response. *Global Health Governance*, 3(2): 1–18.

Katz R and Singer DA (2007) Health and Security in Foreign Policy. *Bulletin of the World Health Organization*, 85(3): 233–4.

Kerr JA (ed) (1970) *Building the Health Bridge: Selections from the Works of Fred L. Soper, M.D.* Bloomington: Indiana University Press.

King NB (2002) Security, Disease, Commerce: Ideologies of Postcolonial Global Health. *Social Studies of Science*, 32(5–6): 763–89.

Klein B (1948) Germany's Preparation for War: A Re-examination. *The American Economic Review*, 38(1): 56–77.

Knudsen O (2001) Post-Copenhagen Security Studies: Desecuritizing Securitization. *Security Dialogue*, 32(3): 355–68.

Koh T, Plant A and Lee EH (eds) (2003) *The New Global Threat: Severe Acute Respiratory Syndrome and Its Impact.* Singapore: World Scientific Publishing.

Kronmen K, Ampofo W, Nzussouo T, Wasfy M, Agbenohevi P, Carroll J, Diabate M, Sourabie S, Puplampu N, Clemens M and Oyofo B (2013) Building Military Influenza Surveillance Capacity in West Africa. *Military Medicine*, 178(3): 306–14.

Kumaresan J, Heitkamp P, Smith I and Billo N (2004) Global Partnership to Stop TB: A Model of an Effective Public Health Partnership. *The International Journal of Tuberculosis and Lung Disease*, 8(1): 120–9.

Lakoff A (2010) Two Regimes of Global Health. *Humanity*, 1(1): 59–79.

Larson JS (1996) The World Health Organization's Definition of Health: Social versus Spiritual Health. *Social Indicators Research*, 38(2): 181–92.

Lauterbach AT (1944) Economic Demobilization in a Conquered Country: Germany 1919–1923. *The Journal of Politics*, 6(1): 28–56.

Lawrence RG (2000) Game-Framing the Issues: Tracking the Strategy Frame in Public Policy News. *Political Communication*, 17(2): 93–114.

Leach-Kemon K, Chou DP, Schneider MT, Tardiff A, Dieleman JL, Brooks B, Hanlon M and Murray C (2012) The Global Financial Crisis has Led to a Slowdown in Growth of Funding to Improve Health in Many Developing Countries. *Health Affairs*, 31(1): 228–35.

League of Nations Health Organization (1931) *Health.* Geneva: League of Nations.

Lederberg J (1996) Infectious Disease – A Threat to Global Health and Security. *Journal of the American Medical Association*, 276(5): 417–19.

Lee K (2003) *Globalization and Health: An Introduction.* Basingstoke: Palgrave Macmillan.

Lee K (2009) *The World Health Organization (WHO).* London: Routledge.

Léonard S and Kaunert C (2011) Reconceptualizing the Audience in Securitization Theory. In Balzacq T (ed) *Securitization Theory: How Security Problems Emerge and Resolve.* Oxon: Routledge: 57–76.

Lerer L and Matzopoulos R (2001) 'The Worst of Both Worlds': The Management Reform of the World Health Organization. *International Journal of Health Services*, 31(2): 415–38.

Lidén J (2014) The World Health Organization and Global Health Governance: Post 1990. *Public Health*, 128(2): 141–7.

Loh C, Galbraith V and Chiu W (2004) The Media and SARS. In Loh C (ed) *At the Epicentre: Hong Kong and the SARS Outbreak*. Hong Kong: Hong Kong University Press: 195–214.

Lowe C (2010) Viral Clouds: Becoming H5N1 in Indonesia. *Cultural Anthropology*, 25(4): 625–49.

Lyne MM, Nielson DL and Tierney MJ (2006) Who Delegates? Alternative Models of Principals in Development Aid. In Hawkins D, Lake D, Nielson D and Tierney M (eds) *Delegation and Agency in International Organizations*. Cambridge: Cambridge University Press: 41–76.

Macfarlane SN (2004) A Useful Concept that Risks Losing Its Political Salience. *Security Dialogue*, 35(3): 368–9.

Mach A (1998) The New WHO Cabinet Looks Refreshingly Different. *BMJ*, 317(7157): 492.

MacKenzie M (1950) International Collaboration in Health. *International Affairs*, 26(4): 515–21.

MacKenzie M (2009) Securitization and Desecuritization: Female Soldiers and the Reconstruction of Women in Post-Conflict Sierra Leone. *Security Studies*, 18(2): 241–61.

Maclean S (2008) Microbes, Mad Cows and Militaries: Exploring the Links Between Health and Security. *Security Dialogue*, 39(5): 475–94.

MacPhail T (2009) The Politics of Bird Flu: The Battle over Virus Samples and China's Role in Global Public Health. *Journal of Language and Politics*, 8(3): 456–75.

Martin R and Conseil S (2012) Public Health Policy and Law for Pandemic Influenza: A Case for European Harmonization? *Journal of Health Politics, Policy and Law*, 37(6): 1089–108.

Martin L and Simmons B (1998) Theories and Empirical Studies of International Institutions. *International Organization*, 52(4): 730–42.

Mason J and Giahyue J (2014) Citing Security Threat, Obama Expands U.S. Role Fighting Ebola. *Reuters*, 16 September 2014. Accessed 8 November 2014. http://www.reuters.com/article/2014/09/16/us-health-ebola-obama-idUSKBN0HB08S20140916

McCormack T (2008) Power and Agency in the Human Security Framework. *Cambridge Review of International Affairs*, 21(1): 113–28.

McDonald M (2008) Securitization and the Construction of Security. *European Journal of International Relations*, 14(4): 563–87.

McDonald M (2011) Deliberation and Resecuritization: Australia, Asylum-Seekers and the Normative Limits of the Copenhagen School. *Australian Journal of Political Science*, 46(2): 281–95.

McInnes C (2015) The Many Meanings of Health Security. In Rushton S and Youde J (eds) *Routledge Handbook of Global Health Security*. Abingdon: Routledge: 7–17.

McInnes C, Kamradt-Scott A, Lee K, Reubi D, Roemer-Mahler A, Rushton S, Williams O and Woodling M (2012) Framing Global Health: The Governance Challenge. *Global Public Health*, 7(Supp 2): S83–94.

McInnes C, Kamradt-Scott A, Lee K, Roemer-Mahler A, Rushton S and Williams O (2014) *The Transformation of Global Health Governance*. London: Palgrave Macmillan.

McInnes C and Lee K (2006) Health, Security and Foreign Policy. *Review of International Studies*, 32(1): 5–23.

McInnes C and Rushton S (2010) HIV, AIDS and Security: Where are We Now? *International Affairs*, 86(1): 225–45.

McNeil D (2009) W.H.O. to Rewrite Its Pandemic Rules. *New York Times*, 23 May 2009, A9.

Mitrany D (1945) "International Public Administration": Problems of International Administration. *Public Administration*, 23(1): 2–12.

Mitrany D (1946) *A Working Peace System: An Argument for the Functional Development of International Organization*. London: National Peace Council.

Mohammadi D (2012) The Final Push for Polio Eradication? *Lancet*, 380(9840): 460–2.

Murphy J and Zhu J (2012) Neo-colonialism in the Academy? Anglo-American Domination in Management Journals. *Organization*, 19(6): 915–27.

Mwacalimba K and Green J (2014) 'One Health' and Development Priorities in Resource-Constrained Countries: Policy Lessons from Avian and Pandemic Influenza Preparedness in Zambia. *Health Policy and Planning*, Published online 14 February 2014, doi:10.1093/heapol/czu001.

Mykhalovskiy E and Weir L (2006) The Global Public Health Intelligence Network and Early Warning Outbreak Detection: A Canadian Contribution to Global Public Health. *Canadian Journal of Public Health*, 97(1): 42–4.

Nabarro D (2014) Phone Interview with Author, 30 May 2014. Sydney, Australia.

Nelson TE (2004) Policy Goals, Public Rhetoric, and Political Attitudes. *Journal of Politics*, 66(2): 581–605.

Nelson TE and Oxley ZM (1999) Issue Framing Effects on Belief Importance and Opinion. *The Journal of Politics*, 61(4): 1040–67.

Nielson DL and Tierney MJ (2003) Delegation to International Organizations: Agency Theory and World Bank Environmental Reform. *International Organization*, 57(2): 241–76.

Nunes J (2014) *Security, Emancipation and the Politics of Health*. Oxon: Routledge.

Nye J (2001) Globalization's Democratic Deficit. *Foreign Affairs*, 80(4): 2–6.

Oestreich J (ed) (2012) *International Organizations as Self-Directed Actors: A Framework for Analysis*. New York: Routledge.

Ollila E (2005) Global Health Priorities – Priorities of the Wealthy? *Globalization and Health*, 1: 6, doi:10.1186/1744-8603-1-6.

Oswald SU (2011) Can Health be Securitized? *Global Bioethics*, 24(1–4): 25–34.

Owens A, Canas L, Russell K, Neville J, Pavlin J, MacIntosh V, Gray G and Gaydos J (2009) Department of Defense Global Laboratory-Based Influenza Surveillance 1998–2005. *American Journal of Preventive Medicine*, 37(3): 235–41.

PAHO (2009a) Influenza Cases by a New Sub-type: Regional Update. *Pan American Health Organization*, 26 April 2009. Accessed 6 May 2014. http://new.paho.org/hq/dmdocuments/2009/epi-alerts-2009-04-26-6pm-swine-flu.pdf

PAHO (2009b) Influenza Cases by a New Sub-type: Regional Update. *Pan American Health Organization*, 28 April 2009. Accessed 6 May 2014. http://new.paho.org/hq/dmdocuments/2009/epi_alerts_2009_04_28_13h_swine_flu.pdf

Paris R (2001) Human Security: Paradigm Shift or Hot Air? *International Security*, 26(2): 87–102.

Parry J (2003a) China Joins Global Effort over Pneumonia Virus. *BMJ*, 326(7393): 781.

Parry J (2003b) China Still not Open Enough about SARS, Says WHO. *BMJ*, 326(7398): 1055.

Payne A (1953) The Influenza Programme of WHO. *Bulletin of the World Health Organization*, 8(5–6): 755–92.

Peabody JW (1995) An Organizational Analysis of the World Health Organization: Narrowing the Gap between Promise and Performance. *Social Science & Medicine*, 40(6): 731–42.

Pereira MS (1979) Global Surveillance of Influenza. *British Medical Bulletin*, 35(1): 9–14.

Phommasack B, Moen A, Vongphrachanh P, Tsuyuoka R, Cox N, Khamphaphongphanh B, Phonekeo D, Kasai T, Ketmayoon P, Lewis H, Kounnavong B, Khanthamalay V and Corwin A (2012) Capacity Building in Response to Pandemic Influenza Threats: Lao PDR Case Study. *American Journal of Tropical Medicine and Hygiene*, 87(6): 965–71.

Piot P (2006) AIDS: From Crisis Management to Sustained Strategic Response. *The Lancet*, 368(9534): 526–30.

Plotkin BJ, Hardiman M, Gonzalez-Martin F and Rodier G (2007) Infectious Disease Surveillance and the International Health Regulations. In M'Inkanantha NM, Lynfield R, Van Beneden CA and de Valk H (eds) *Infectious Disease Surveillance*. Massachusetts: Blackwell Publishing: 18–31.

Poku N, Whiteside A and Sandkjaer B (eds) (2007) *AIDS and Governance (Global Health)*. Hampshire: Ashgate.

Porter D (1999) *Health, Civilization and the State: A History of Public Health from Ancient to Modern Times*. London: Routledge.

Porter D (2006) How Did Social Medicine Evolve, and Where is It Heading? *PLoS Medicine*, 3: e999. doi:10.1371/journal.pmed.0030399.

Pratt D (1999) Lessons for Implementation from the World's Most Successful Programme: The Global Eradication of Smallpox. *Journal of Curriculum Studies*, 31(2): 177–94.

Pyhälä R (1980) Protection by a Polyvalent Influenza Vaccine and Persistence of Homologous and Heterologous H1 Antibodies during a Period of Two Epidemic Seasons. *Journal of Hygiene Cambridge*, 84(2): 237–45.

Raufu A (2004a) Nigeria Postpones Programme of Polio Immunisation. *BMJ*, 328(7451): 1278.

Raufu A (2004b) Traditional Rulers in Northern Nigeria Call for Halt to Polio Vaccination. *BMJ*, 328(7435): 306–7.

Raviglione MC, Dye C, Schmidt S and Kochi A (1997) Assessment of Worldwide Tuberculosis Control. *The Lancet*, 350(9078): 624–9.

Raviglione MC and Pio A (2002) Evolution of WHO Policies for Tuberculosis Control, 1948–2001. *The Lancet*, 359(9308): 775–80.

Rein M and Schön DA (1993) Reframing Policy Discourse. In Fischer F and Duke F (eds) *The Argumentative Turn in Policy Analysis and Planning*. London: University Press: 145–66.

Riccardi G, Pasca MR and Buroni S (2009) Mycobacterium Tuberculosis: Drug Resistance and Future Perspectives. *Future Microbiology*, 4(5): 597–614.

Rochester JM (1986) The Rise and Fall of International Organization as a Field of Study. *International Organization*, 40(4): 777–813.

Roden A (1963) Influenza as a National Problem. *Postgraduate Medical Journal*, 39(456): 612–18.

Rodier G (2003) Why was Toronto Included in the World Health Organization's SARS-Related Travel Advisory?. *CMAJ*, 168(11): 1434–5.

Rodier G (2009) Personal Interview with Author, 16 June 2009. Geneva: Switzerland.

Rodier G, Greenspan A, Hughes J and Heymann D (2007) Global Public Health Security. *Emerging Infectious Diseases*, 13(10): 1447–52.

Roe P (2004) Securitization and Minority Rights: Conditions of Desecuritization. *Security Dialogue*, 35(3): 279–94.

Roe P (2012) Is Securitization a 'Negative' Concept? Revisiting the Normative Debate over Normal versus Extraordinary Politics. *Security Dialogue*, 43(3): 249–66.

Rushton S (2011) Global Health Security: Security for Whom? Security from What? *Political Studies*, 59(4): 779–96.

Rushton S (2012) The Global Debate Over HIV-Related Travel Restrictions: Framing and Policy Change. *Global Public Health*, 7(Supp 2): S159–75.

Ruxin J, Paluzzi JE, Wilson PA, Tozan Y, Kruk M and Teklehaimanot A (2005) Emerging Consensus in HIV/AIDS, Malaria, Tuberculosis, and Access to Essential Medicines. *The Lancet*, 365(9459): 618–21.

Ryan M (2009) Telephone Interview with Author, 24 June 2009. London.

Saengdidtha B and Rangsin R (2005) Roles of the Royal Thai Army Medical Department in Supporting the Country to Fight against HIV/AIDS: 18 Years of Experience and Success. *Journal of the Medical Association of Thailand*, 88 (Supp 3): S378–86.

Salter MB (2008) Securitization and Desecuritization: A Dramaturgical Analysis of the Canadian Air Transport Security Authority. *Journal of International Relations and Development*, 11(4): 321–49.

Sands P and Klein P (2001) *Bowett's Law of International Institutions*. 5th edition. London: Sweet and Maxwell.

Sangeeta S (2007) WHO Meeting on Avian Flu Virus Ends with Draft Documents. *Third World Network*, 28 November. Accessed 18 July 2014. http://www.twnside. org.sg/title2/health.info/twnhealthinfo041107.htm

Sarooshi D (2005) *International Organizations and Their Exercise of Sovereign Powers*. Oxford: Oxford University Press.

Sawyer WA (1947) Achievements of UNRRA as an International Health Organization. *American Journal of Public Health*, 37(1): 41–58.

Schermers HG and Blokker NM (2003) *International Institutional Law*. 4th revised edition. Boston: Martinus Nijhoff.

Schlein L (2003) Refusal of Polio Vaccines in Nigeria Could Have Tragic Consequences, Warns WHO. *Voice of America*. Accessed 28 July 2014. http:// www.voanews.com/content/a-13-a-2003-10-31-38-refusal/392752.html

Seckinelgin H (2012) *International Security, Conflict and Gender: 'HIV/AIDS is Another War'*. London: Routledge.

Sedyaningsih ER, Isfandari S, Soendoro T and Supari SF (2008) Towards Mutual Trust, Transparency and Equity in Virus Sharing Mechanism: The Avian Influenza Case of Indonesia. *Annuals of the Academy of Medicine, Singapore*, 37(6): 482–8.

Selgelid M and Enemark C (2008) Infectious Diseases, Security and Ethics: The Case of HIV/AIDS. *Bioethics*, 22(9): 457–65.

Sharp WR (1947) The New World Health Organization. *American Journal of International Law*, 41: 509–30.

Shiffman J (2009) A Social Explanation for the Rise and Fall of Global Health Issues. *Bulletin of the World Health Organization*, 87(8): 608–13.

Shkabatur J (2011) A Global Panopticon? The Changing Role of International Organizations in the Information Age. *Michigan Journal of International Law*, 33: 159–214.

Shuchman M (2007) Improving Global Health-Margaret Chan at the WHO. *New England Journal of Medicine*, 356(7): 653–6.

Siddiqi J (1995) *World Health and World Politics: The World Health Organization and the U.N. System*. London: Hurst and Company.

Smith A (1992) Military Medicine: Not the Same as Practicing Medicine in the Military. *Armed Forces & Society*, 18(4): 576–91.

Smith K (2013a) Institutional Filters: The Translation and Re-circulation of Ideas about Health Inequalities within Policy. *Policy & Politics*, 41(1): 81–100.

Smith J (2013b) A Critique of the Response by Global Health Initiatives to HIV/AIDS in Africa: Implications for Countries Emerging from Conflict. *International Peacekeeping*, 20(4): 536–50.

Smith III F (2014) *American Biodefense: How Dangerous Ideas About Biological Weapons Shape National Security*. Ithaca: Cornell University Press.

Smith W, Andrewes C and Laidlaw P (1933) A Virus Obtained from Influenza Patients. *Lancet*, 222(5732): 66–8.

Snacken R, Kendal A, Haaheim L and Wood J (1999) The Next Influenza Pandemic: Lessons from Hong Kong, 1997. *Emerging Infectious Diseases*, 5(2): 195–203.

SooHoo C (2009) WHO to Revise Definition of Pandemic Phases Amidst 2009 H1N1 Pandemic. *Biosecurity and Bioterrorism*, 7(2): 117–18.

Sridhar D, Frenk J, Gostin L and Moon S (2014) Global Rules for Global Health: Why We Need an Independent, Impartial WHO. *BMJ*, 348: g3841. doi:http://dx.doi.org/10.1136/bmj.g3841

Sridhar D and Gostin L (2011) Reforming the World Health Organization. *JAMA*, 305(15): 1585–6.

Stapleton D (2004) Lessons of History? Anti-malaria Strategies of the International Health Board and the Rockefeller Foundation from the 1920s to the Era of DDT. *Public Health Chronicles*, 119(2): 206–15.

Stephenson N (2012) The Disappearing Act of Global Health Security. In Enemark C and Selgelid M (eds) *Ethics and Security Aspects of Infectious Disease Control: Interdisciplinary Perspectives*. Surrey: Ashgate: 97–110.

Stevenson M and Moran M (2015) Health Security and the Distortion of the Global Health Agenda. In Rushton S and Youde J (eds) *Routledge Handbook of Global Health Security*. Abingdon: Routledge: 328–38.

Stewart W (1958) Administrative History of the Asian Influenza Program. *Public Health Reports (1896–1970)*, 73(2): 101–13.

Stewart P (2014) UPDATE 1-U.S. Ramps up Ebola Troop Deployments, Total May Near 4,000. *Reuters*, 3 October 2014. Accessed 8 November 2014. http://www.reuters.com/article/2014/10/03/health-ebola-usa-pentagon-idUSL2N0RY1TH20141003

Stöhr K (2003a) A Multicentre Collaboration to Investigate the Cause of Severe Acute Respiratory Syndrome. *The Lancet*, 361(9370): 1730–3.

Stöhr K (2003b) The Global Agenda on Influenza Prevention and Control. *Vaccine*, 21(16): 1744–8.

Stone RW (2008) The Scope of IMF Conditionality. *International Organization*, 62(4): 589–620.

Stop TB Partnership (2001) *Global Plan to Stop TB, Phase 1: 2001–2005*. Geneva: World Health Organization.

Stop TB Partnership (2004) *Basic Framework for the Global Partnership to Stop TB*. Geneva: Stop TB Partnership Secretariat.

Stop TB Partnership (2006) *The Global Plan to Stop TB, 2006–2015. Actions for Life: Towards a World Free of Tuberculosis*. Geneva: World Health Organization.

Stowman K (1952) International Sanitary Regulations. *Public Health Reports*, 67(10): 972–6.

Stritzel H (2007) Towards a Theory of Securitization: Copenhagen and Beyond. *European Journal of International Relations*, 13(3): 357–83.

Sydenstricker E (1924) Current World Prevalence of Disease: Review of the Monthly Epidemiological Report for 15 June 1924, Issued by the Health Section of the League of Nations' Secretariat. *Public Health Reports (1896–1970)*, 39(31): 1842–5.

Tan Y (2003) Combating SARS with Infrared Fever Screening System (IFSS). In Koh T, Plant A and Lee E (eds) *The New Global Threat: Severe Acute Respiratory Syndrome and Its Impacts*. Singapore: World Scientific: 283–300.

Tan D, Upshur R and Ford N (2003) Global Plagues and the Global Fund: Challenges in the Fight against HIV/AIDS, TB and Malaria. *BMC International Health and Human Rights*, 3(2): 1–9.

Tayob RK (2008) WHO Board Debates "Global Health Security", Climate, IPRs. *Third World Network*, Geneva: Switzerland. Accessed 24 July 2014. www.twnside.org.sg/title2/health.info/2008/twnhealthinfo010108.htm

Thomson E and Yow C (2004) The Hong Kong SAR Government, Civil Society and SARS. In Wong J and Zheng Y (eds) *The SARS Epidemic: Challenges to China's Crisis Management*. Singapore: World Scientific: 199–220.

Tren R and Bate R (2001) *Malaria and the DDT Story*. London: Institute of Economic Affairs.

Tucker B (1999) From Arms Race to Abolition: The Evolving Norm against Biological and Chemical Warfare. In Drell S, Sofaer A and Wilson G (eds) *The New Terror: Facing the Threat of Biological and Chemical Weapons*. Stanford: Hoover Institution Press: 159-226.

UK Government (2008) *Health is Global: A UK Government Strategy 2008–13*. London: HM Government.

UN (2014a) Avian Influenza and the Pandemic Threat: About UNSIC. Accessed 28 May 2014. http://www.un-influenza.org/?q=content/about-unsic

UN (2014b) Resolution 2177(2014). Accessed 8 November 2014. http://www.un.org/en/ga/search/view_doc.asp?symbol=S/RES/2177%20%282014%29

UN (2014c) UN Mission for Ebola Emergency Response (UNMEER). Accessed 10 November 2014. http://www.un.org/ebolaresponse/mission.shtml

UNAIDS (2008) *UNAIDS: The First 10 Years*. Geneva: Joint United Nations Programme on HIV/AIDS.

UNDP (1994) *Human Development Report 1994: New Dimensions of Human Security*. Oxford: Oxford University Press.

UNSIC (2006) Avian and Human Influenza (AHI): Consolidated Action Plan for Contributions of the UN System and Partners: Revised Activities and Financial Requirements up to December 2007. New York: United Nations System Influenza Coordinator. Accessed 5 June 2014. http://www.un-influenza.org/sites/default/files/review_nov06_dec07.pdf

US GAO (2004) *Emerging Infectious Diseases: Asian SARS Outbreak Challenged International and National Responses*. Washington, DC: United States General Accounting Office. Accessed 26 July 2014. http://www.gao.gov/products/GAO-04-564

van de Pas R and van Schaik LG (2014) Democratizing the World Health Organization. *Public Health*, 128(2): 195–201.

Vaughan JP, Mogedal S, Kruse SE, Lee K, Walt G and de Wilde K (1995) *Cooperation for Health Development: Extrabudgetary Funds in the World Health Organization* (Joint publication by the Australian Agency for International Development, the Norwegian Royal Ministry of Foreign Affairs, and the United Kingdom Overseas Development Administration).

Velimirovic B (1976) Do We Still Need International Health Regulations? *The Journal of Infectious Diseases*, 133(4): 478–81.

Vuori JA (2008) Illocutionary Logic and Strands of Securitization: Applying the Theory of Securitization to the Study of Non-Democratic Political Orders. *European Journal of International Relations*, 14(1): 65–99.

Wæver O (1995) Securitization and Desecuritization. In Lipschultz R (ed) *On Security*. New York: Colombia University Press: 46–86.

Wæver O (2011) Politics, Security, Theory. *Security Dialogue*, 42(4–5): 465–80.

Walters JH (1978) Influenza 1918: The Contemporary Perspective. *Bulletin of the New York Academy of Medicine*, 54(9): 855–64.

Watterson S and Kamradt-Scott A (2015) Fighting Flu: Securitization and the Military Role in Combatting Influenza. *Armed Forces & Society*, first published on 20 January 2015 as doi:10.1177/0095327X14567364

Watson S (2012) 'Framing' the Copenhagen School: Integrating the Literature on Threat Construction. *Millennium*, 40(2): 279–301.

Weaver C (2007) The World's Bank and the Bank's World. *Global Governance*, 13(4): 493–512.

Webster R (1994) While Awaiting the Next Pandemic of Influenza. *BMJ*, 309(6063): 1179.

Webster R and Kawaoka Y (1994) Influenza – An Emerging and Re-emerging Disease. *Virology*, 5(2): 103–11. (Ch. 5, p. 7).

Weir L (2015) Inventing Global Health Security, 1994–2005. In Rushton S and Youde J (eds) *Routledge Handbook of Global Health Security*. Abingdon: Routledge: 18–31.

Whelan M (2008) *Negotiating the International Health Regulations*. Global Health Working Paper No. 1. Geneva: Graduate Institute.

Whelan M (2009) Telephone Interview with Author, 2 June 2009. London.

WHO (1947a) Minutes of the Technical Preparatory Committee for the International Health Conference, Held in Paris from 18 March to 5 April 1946. *Official Records of the World Health Organization*. No. 1.

WHO (1947b) *Chronicle of the World Health Organization: Development and Constitution of the WHO.* 1(1–2).

WHO (1947c) *Official Records of the World Health Organization.* No. 4. Geneva: World Health Organization.

WHO (1948a) *Chronicle of the World Health Organization.* 2(1). Geneva: World Health Organization.

WHO (1948b) *Official Records of the World Health Organization.* No. 2. Geneva: World Health Organization.

WHO (1948c) *Official Records of the World Health Organization.* No. 10. Geneva: World Health Organization.

WHO (1948d) *Official Records of the World Health Organization.* No. 6. Geneva: World Health Organization.

WHO (1951) *International Sanitary Regulations: World Health Organization Regulations No. 2.* Technical Report Series No. 41. Geneva: World Health Organization.

WHO (1953) *Expert Committee on Influenza: First Report. World Health Organization Technical Report Series No. 64.* Geneva: World Health Organization.

WHO (1955) *Official Records of the World Health Organization.* No. 63. Geneva: World Health Organization.

WHO (1956a) Report on the Inter-Regional Conference on Malaria and on the Expert Committee of Malaria (6th Session) Convened by the World Health Organization in Athens (Greece) in June, 1956. M_2/81/6(b). (Malaria Archive).

WHO (1957a) Annex 11: Malaria Eradication – Report on Implementation of Resolutions WHA8.30 and WHA9.61. *Official Records of the World Health Organization.* No. 79. Geneva: World Health Organization.

WHO (1957b) Review of Work during 1956: Annual Report of the Director-General. *Official Records of the World Health Organization,* 79: 182–256.

WHO (1958) *The First Ten Years of the World Health Organization.* Geneva: World Health Organization.

WHO (1959a) *Official Record of the World Health Organization.* No. 87. Geneva: World Health Organization.

WHO (1959b) *Expert Committee on Respiratory Viruses: First Report. World Health Organization Technical Report Series No. 170.* Geneva: World Health Organization.

WHO (1960a) Progress of Malaria Projects in the Western Pacific Region. Mal/Exp.Com.8/WP/22. (Malaria Archive).

WHO (1960b) The Use of Drugs in Malaria Eradication Programmes. Mal/Exp.Com.8/WP/24, pp. 1–7. (Malaria Archive).

WHO (1960c) Cycles and Dosages of Insecticides in Eradication Programmes. Document: Mal/Exp.Com.8/WP/33. (WHO Archive).

WHO (1960d) *Expert Committee on Tuberculosis: Seventh Report.* Technical Report Series No. 195. Geneva: World Health Organization.

WHO (1962) *Official Record of the World Health Organization.* No. 111. Geneva: World Health Organization.

WHO (1965a) Annex 11: Development of the Malaria Eradication Programme. *Official Records of the World Health Organization.* No. 143. Geneva: World Health Organization.

WHO (1965b) Annex 19: Smallpox Eradication Programme. *Official Records of the World Health Organization.* No. 143: 161–75.

WHO (1966a) Smallpox Eradication (Proposed Method of Financing): Report by the Director-General. EB37/23_Add.1.

WHO (1966b) Minutes of the Ninth Meeting. EB/37/Min/9_Rev.1.

WHO (1966c) Preparation for the Implementation of the Smallpox Eradication Programme. Memorandum dated 6 June 1966. Smallpox Archive, Box 3, ID 27. Geneva: World Health Organization.

WHO (1966d) Paper by Dr Bland – Observations on the Inter-relationship between Smallpox Eradication and Public Health Services. Smallpox Archive, Box 3, ID 27. Geneva: World Health Organization.

WHO (1966e) Paper prepared by Dr Karel Raska – Global Eradication of Smallpox. Smallpox Archive, Box 3, ID 27. Geneva: World Health Organization.

WHO (1967a) *WHO Expert Committee on Malaria: Thirteenth Report*. Technical Report Series No. 357. Geneva: World Health Organization.

WHO (1967b) *Handbook for Smallpox Eradication Programmes in Endemic Areas*. Geneva: World Health Organization.

WHO (1968a) *The Second Ten Years of the World Health Organization, 1958–1967*. Geneva: World Health Organization.

WHO (1968b) Surveillance – The Key to Smallpox Eradication. WHO/SE/68.2.

WHO (1968c) *Smallpox Eradication: Report of a WHO Scientific Group. World Health Organization Technical Report Series No. 393*. Geneva: World Health Organization.

WHO (1969a) Annex 13: Re-examination of the Global Strategy of Malaria Eradication. *Official Record of the World Health Organization*. No. 176. Geneva: World Health Organization.

WHO (1969b) *Respiratory Viruses: Report of a WHO Scientific Group*. Technical Report Series No. 408. Geneva: World Health Organization.

WHO (1970) *Insecticide Resistance and Vector Control: 17th Report of the WHO Expert Committee on Insecticides*. Technical Report Series No. 443. Geneva: World Health Organization.

WHO (1973) *Handbook of the Resolutions and Decisions of the World Health Assembly and Executive Board, Volume 1, 1948–1972*. Geneva: World Health Organization.

WHO (1988) Consultation with Directors of WHO Collaborating Centres on Influenza: Memorandum from a WHO Meeting. *Bulletin of the World Health Organization*, 66(4): 457–8.

WHO (1993a) *Handbook of Resolutions and Decisions of the World Health Assembly and Executive Board. Volume III, Third Edition (1985–1992)*. Geneva: World Health Organization.

WHO (1993b) *Forty-Sixth World Health Assembly*. Geneva, 3–14 May 1993. Resolutions and Decisions, Annexes. WHA46/1993/REC/1.

WHO (1994) WHO Tuberculosis Programme: Framework for Effective Tuberculosis Control. WHO/TB/94.179.

WHO (1996a) *World Health Report, 1996: Fighting Disease, Fostering Development*. Geneva: World Health Organization.

WHO (1996b) The International Response to Epidemics and Applications of the International Health Regulations: Report of a WHO Informal Consultation. WHO/EMC/IHR/96.1. Accessed 8 July 2014. http://whqlibdoc.who.int/hq/1996/WHO_EMC_IHR_96.1.pdf

WHO (1998a) Address to WHO Staff. Accessed 9 May 2005. http://www.who.int/director-general/speeches/1998/english/19980721_bg_staff.html

WHO (1998b) *Fifty Years of the World Health Organization in the Western Pacific Region, 1948–1998*. Manilla: Western Pacific Regional Office.

WHO (1998c) The World Health Report 1998. Life in the 21st Century: A Vision for All: Summary. Provisional Agenda Item 10, A51/3. Accessed 19 May 2014. http://apps.who.int/iris/bitstream/10665/79737/1/ea3.pdf?ua=1

WHO (1999a) Looking Ahead for WHO after a Year of Change: Statement by the Director-General to the Fifty-Second World Health Assembly. A52/3. Geneva: World Health Organization.

WHO (1999b) *Influenza Pandemic Preparedness Plan: The Role of WHO and Guidelines for National and Regional Planning*. Geneva: World Health Organization.

WHO (2000a) *A Framework for Global Outbreak Alert and Response*. Geneva: World Health Organization.

WHO (2000b) An Integrated Approach to Communicable Disease Surveillance. *Weekly Epidemiological Record*, 75(1): 1–7.

WHO (2000c) *Global Outbreak Alert and Response. Report of a WHO Meeting*. Geneva: World Health Organization.

WHO (2000d) *WHO Report on Global Surveillance of Epidemic-prone Infectious Diseases*. Geneva: World Health Organization.

WHO (2000e) Revision of the International Health Regulations: Progress Report, July 2000. *Weekly Epidemiological Record*, 75(29): 234–6.

WHO (2000f) *Global Outbreak Alert and Response. Report of a WHO Meeting*. Geneva: World Health Organization.

WHO (2001a) WHA54.14 Global Health Security: Epidemic Alert and Response, 21 May 2001. Accessed 26 July 2014. http://apps.who.int/gb/archive/pdf_files/WHA54/ea54r14.pdf

WHO (2001b) Provisional Summary Record of the Eighth Meeting, Committee A, Fifty-Fourth World Health Assembly. A54/A/SR/8.

WHO (2001c) Revision of the International Health Regulations: Progress Report, February 2001. *Weekly Epidemiological Record*, 76(8): 61–3.

WHO (2001d) Global Health Security – Epidemic Alert and Response: Report by the Secretariat. A54/9. Accessed 19 May 2014. http://apps.who.int/gb/archive/pdf_files/WHA54/ea549.pdf

WHO (2002a) *Tuberculosis: Epidemiology and Control*. Geneva: World Health Organization.

WHO (2002b) *Preparedness for the Deliberate Use of Biological Agents: A Rational Approach to the Unthinkable*. Geneva: World Health Organization.

WHO (2002c) Revision of the International Health Regulations: Progress Report, May 2002. *Weekly Epidemiological Record*, 77(19): 158–9.

WHO (2003a) *!Outbreak: Global Health Security from the World Health Organization*. Geneva: World Health Organization.

WHO (2003b) WHO Issues a Global Alert About Cases of Atypical Pneumonia: Cases of Severe Respiratory Illness May Spread to Hospital Staff. Accessed 26 July 2014. http://www.who.int/mediacentre/news/releases/2003/pr22/en/

WHO (2003c) Revision of the International Health Regulations: Severe Acute Respiratory Syndrome (SARS). Report by the Secretariat. A56/48.

WHO (2003d) Influenza A(H5N1) in Hong Kong Special Administrative Region of China – Update. Accessed 26 July 2014. http://www.who.int/csr/don/2003_02_20/en

WHO (2003e) The Operational Response to SARS. Accessed 26 July 2014. http://www.who.int/csr/sars/goarn2003_4_16/en/

WHO (2003f) WHO Recommended Measures for Persons Undertaking International Travel from Areas Affected by Severe Acute Respiratory Syndrome (SARS). *Weekly Epidemiological Record*, 78(14): 98–9.

WHO (2003g) Hospital Infection Control Guidance for Severe Acute Respiratory Syndrome (SARS). Accessed 26 July 2014. http://www.who.int/ihr/lyon/surveillance/infectioncontrol/en/

WHO (2003h) Severe Acute Respiratory Syndrome (SARS) Multi-country Outbreak – Update 3. Accessed 26 July 2014. http://www.who.int/csr/don/2003_03_18/en/index.html

WHO (2003i) SARS outbreak: WHO Investigation Team Moves to Guangdong China, New Travel Advice Announced. Accessed 26 July 2014. http://www.who.int/mediacentre/news/releases/2003/pr29/en/

WHO (2003j) Update 40 – Situation in Shanghai, Hong Kong and Vietnam. Accessed 26 July 2014. http://www.who.int/csr/sarsarchive/2003_04_26/en

WHO (2003k) WHO Frontline Worker Dies of Severe Acute Respiratory Syndrome (SARS). *Bulletin of the World Health Organization*, 81(5): 384.

WHO (2003l) Severe Acute Respiratory Syndrome – Virtual Press Briefing. Accessed 26 July 2014. http://www.who.int/csr/sars/2003_04_25/en/

WHO (2003m) WHA56.28 Revision of the International Health Regulations. Accessed 27 July 2014. http://apps.who.int/gb/archive/pdf_files/WHA56/ea56r28.pdf

WHO (2004a) Consultation on the Revision of the International Health Regulations (IHR) in the Western Pacific Region. (WP) ICP/CSR/1.1/001.

WHO (2004b) International Health Regulations: Working Paper for Regional Consultations. IGWG/IHR/Working Paper/12.2003.

WHO (2005a) *Basic Documents. Forty-Fifth Edition*. Geneva: World Health Organization.

WHO (2005b) *Global Consultation on Strengthening National Capacities for Surveillance and Control of Communicable Diseases*. Geneva: World Health Organization.

WHO (2005c) Avian Influenza: Frequently Asked Questions. *Weekly Epidemiological Record*, 80(44): 377–88.

WHO (2005d) *Avian Influenza and Human Pandemic Influenza: Summary Report. Meeting Held in Geneva, Switzerland, 7–9 November 2005*. Geneva: World Health Organization. Accessed 3 June 2014. https://extranet.who.int/iris/restricted/bitstream/10665/69216/1/AVIAN_INFLUENZA_sum_report_Nov_05_meeting.pdf

WHO (2005e) Strengthening Pandemic-Influenza Preparedness and Response: Report by the Secretariat. EB117/5. Accessed 3 June 2014. http://apps.who.int/gb/archive/pdf_files/EB117/B117_5-en.pdf

WHO (2005f) *WHO Global Influenza Preparedness Plan: The Role of WHO and Recommendations for National Measures Before and During Pandemics*. Geneva: World Health Organization.

WHO (2006a) *SARS: How a Global Epidemic Was Stopped*. Geneva: World Health Organization.

WHO (2006b) Epidemiology of WHO-Confirmed Human Cases of Avian Influenza A(H5N1) Infection. *Weekly Epidemiological Record*, 81(26): 249–60.

WHO (2006c) *Fifty-Ninth World Health Assembly. Geneva, 22–27 May 2006. Resolutions and Decisions. Annexes.* Geneva: World Health Organization. Accessed 4 June 2014. http://apps.who.int/gb/ebwha/pdf_files/WHA59-REC1/e/WHA59_2006_REC1-en.pdf

WHO (2006d) *WHO Influenza Pandemic Task Force: Report of the First Meeting.* WHO/CDS/EPR/GIP/2006.5. Geneva: World Health Organization.

WHO (2006e) *Engaging for Health: Eleventh General Programme of Work 2006–2015: A Global Health Agenda.* Geneva: World Health Organization. Accessed 18 July 2014. http://whqlibdoc.who.int/publications/2006/GPW_eng.pdf

WHO (2007a) *The World Health Report 2007: A Safer Future: Global Public Health Security in the 21st Century.* Geneva: World Health Organization.

WHO (2007b) *Putting People and Health Needs on the Map.* Geneva: World Health Organization.

WHO (2007c) Global Outbreak Alert and Response Network – GOARN: Partnership in Outbreak Response. Accessed 8 April 2014. http://www.who.int/csr/outbreaknetwork/goarnenglish.pdf

WHO (2007d) International Spread of Disease Threatens Public Health Security. WHO News Release, 23 August 2007. Accessed 8 April 2014. http://www.who.int/mediacentre/news/releases/2007/pr44/en/

WHO (2007e) Avian and Pandemic Influenza: Developments, Response and Follow-up: Report by the Secretariat. A60/7. Accessed 5 June 2014. http://apps.who.int/gb/ebwha/pdf_files/WHA60/A60_7-en.pdf

WHO (2008a) *The Third Ten Years of the World Health Organization: 1968–1977.* Geneva: World Health Organization.

WHO (2008b) *International Health Regulations (2005).* 2nd edition. Geneva: World Health Organization.

WHO (2008c) Pandemic Influenza Preparedness: Sharing of Influenza Viruses and Access to Vaccines and Other Benefits: Intergovernmental Meeting: Progress to Date. EB122/5. Accessed 5 June 2014. http://apps.who.int/gb/ebwha/pdf_files/EB122/B122_5-en.pdf

WHO (2008d) *WHO-China Country Cooperation Strategy, 2008–2013.* Geneva: World Health Organization. Accessed 18 July 2014. http://s3.documentcloud.org/documents/365336/who-china-country-cooperation-strategy-2008-2013.pdf

WHO (2009a) New Influenza A(H1N1) Virus Infections: Global Surveillance Summary, May 2009. *Weekly Epidemiological Record,* 20(84): 173–8.

WHO (2009b) WHO Ad Hoc Scientific Teleconference on the Current Influenza A(H1N1) Situation, 29 April 2009. Accessed 27 July 2014. http://www.who.int/csr/resources/publications/swineflu/TCReport2009_05_04.pdf

WHO (2009c) Influenza A(H1N1) – Update 5, 29 April 2009. Accessed 27 July 2014. http://www.who.int/csr/don/2009_04_29/en/index.html

WHO (2009d) *Pandemic Influenza Preparedness and Response: A WHO Guidance Document.* Geneva: World Health Organization.

WHO (2009e) *Summary Report of a High-Level Consultation: New Influenza A (H1N1). Geneva, 18 May 2009.* Information Note/2009/2, 20 May 2009. Accessed 27 July 2014. http://www.who.int/csr/resources/publications/swineflu/High_Level_Consultation_18_May_2009.pdf

WHO (2009f) Human Infection with New Influenza A (H1N1) Virus: Mexico, Update, March–May 2009. *Weekly Epidemiological Record,* 84(23): 213–48.

WHO (2009g) Third Meeting of the IHR Emergency Committee. Accessed 27 July 2014. http://www.who.int/csr/disease/swineflu/3rd_meeting_ihr/en/index.html

WHO (2009h) Infection Prevention and Control During Health Care for Confirmed, Probable, or Suspected Cases of Pandemic (H1N1) 2009 Virus Infection and Influenza-like Illnesses. Accessed 23 June 2014. http://www.who.int/csr/resources/publications/cp150_2009_1612_ipc_interim_guidance_h1n1.pdf?ua=1

WHO (2009i) Human Infection with New Influenza A (H1N1) Virus: Clinical Observations from Mexico and Other Affected Countries, May 2009. *Weekly Epidemiological Record*, 84(21): 185–96.

WHO (2009j) Swine Influenza – Update 3. Accessed 22 June 2014. http://www.who.int/csr/don/2009_04_27/en/

WHO (2009k) WHO Recommendations on Pandemic (H1N1) 2009 Vaccines. Accessed 23 June 2014. http://www.who.int/csr/disease/swineflu/notes/h1n1_vaccine_20090713/en/

WHO (2009l) Pandemic (H1N1) 2009 Briefing Note 1 Viruses Resistant to Oseltamivir (Tamiflu) Identified. *Weekly Epidemiological Record*, 84(29): 299–300.

WHO (2009m) Human Infection with Pandemic (H1N1) 2009 Virus: Updated Interim WHO Guidance on Global Surveillance. Accessed 23 June 2014. http://www.who.int/csr/disease/swineflu/guidance/surveillance/WHO_case_definition_swine_flu_2009_04_29.pdf

WHO (2009n) Behavioural Interventions for Reducing the Transmission and Impact of Influenza A (H1n1) Virus: A Framework for Communication Strategies. Accessed 23 June 2014. http://www.who.int/csr/resources/publications/swineflu/framework_20090626_en.pdf

WHO (2009o) Reducing Transmission of Pandemic (H1N1) 2009 in School Settings: A Framework for National and Local Planning and Response. Accessed 23 June 2014. http://www.who.int/csr/resources/publications/reducing_transmission_h1n1_2009.pdf

WHO (2009p) New Influenza A (H1N1) Virus: WHO Guidance on Public Health Measures, 11 June 2009. *Weekly Epidemiological Record*, 84(26): 261–8.

WHO (2009q) Patient Care Checklist: New Influenza A (H1N1). Accessed 23 June 2014. http://www.who.int/csr/resources/publications/swineflu/ah1n1_checklist.pdf

WHO (2009r) Joint WHO-OFFLU Technical Teleconference to Discuss Human-Animal Interface Aspects of the Current Influenza A (H1N1) Situation. Accessed 23 June 2014. http://www.who.int/csr/resources/publications/swineflu/WHO_OFFLU2009_05_15.pdf?ua=1

WHO (2009s) Call to Action from WHO, IFRC, UNSIC, OCHA and UNICEF. Accessed 23 June 2014. http://www.who.int/csr/resources/publications/swineflu/20090817_call_to_action_en.pdf

WHO (2009t) H1N1 Influenza Situation: Statement Made at the Secretary-General's Briefing to the United Nations General Assembly on the H1N1 Influenza Situation, 4 May 2009. Accessed 23 June 2014. http://www.who.int/dg/speeches/2009/influenza_a_h1n1_situation_20090504/en/

WHO (2009u) WHO Welcomes Sanofi-Aventis's Donation of Vaccine. Accessed 23 June 2014. http://www.who.int/mediacentre/news/statements/2009/vaccine_donation_20090617/en/

WHO (2009v) Joint FAO/WHO/OIE Statement on Influenza A(H1N1) and the Safety of Pork. Accessed 23 June 2014. http://www.who.int/mediacentre/news/statements/2009/h1n1_20090430/en/

WHO (2010a) H1N1 in Post-pandemic Period. Accessed 23 June 2014. http://www.who.int/mediacentre/news/statements/2010/h1n1_vpc_20100810/en/index.html

WHO (2010b) Statement of the World Health Organization on Allegations of Conflict of Interest and 'Fake' Pandemic. Accessed 27 July 2014. http://www.who.int/mediacentre/news/statements/2010/h1n1_pandemic_20100122/en/

WHO (2010c) *Towards Universal Access: Scaling up Priority HIV/AIDS Interventions in the Health Sector: Progress Report 2010*. Geneva: World Health Organization. Accessed 18 July 2014. http://apps.who.int/iris/bitstream/10665/44443/1/9789241500395_eng.pdf?ua=1

WHO (2011a) *The Fourth Ten Years of the World Health Organization: 1978–1987*. Geneva: World Health Organization.

WHO (2011b) H5N1 Avian Influenza: Timeline of Major Events. Accessed 27 May 2014. http://www.who.int/influenza/human_animal_interface/avian_influenza/H5N1_avian_influenza_update.pdf

WHO (2011c) Director-General Responds to Assessment of WHO's Handling of the Influenza Pandemic. Remarks at the Fourth Meeting of the Review Committee of the International Health Regulations. Accessed 27 July 2014. http://www.who.int/dg/speeches/2011/ihr_review_20110328/en/

WHO (2011d) The Future Financing for WHO: World Health Organization: Reforms for a Healthy Future: Report by the Director-General: Executive Summary. A64/4. Accessed 19 July 2014. http://apps.who.int/gb/ebwha/pdf_files/WHA64/A64_4-en.pdf

WHO (2012a) Implementation of the International Health Regulations (2005): Report by the Director-General. A65/17. Accessed 7 July 2014. http://apps.who.int/gb/ebwha/pdf_files/WHA65/A65_17-en.pdf

WHO (2012b) Implementation of the International Health Regulations (2005): Report on Development of National Core Capacities Required Under the Regulations: Report by the Director-General. A65/17_Add.1. Accessed 7 July 2014. http://apps.who.int/gb/ebwha/pdf_files/WHA65/A65_17Add1-en.pdf

WHO (2012c) WHO Reform: Draft Twelfth Programme of Work and Explanatory Notes. A65/5_Add.1. Accessed 19 July 2014. http://apps.who.int/gb/ebwha/pdf_files/WHA65/A65_5Add1-en.pdf

WHO (2012d) Implementation of the International Health Regulations (2005): Report by the Secretariat. A65/17. Accessed 19 July 2014. http://apps.who.int/gb/ebwha/pdf_files/WHA65/A65_17-en.pdf

WHO (2012e) Pandemic Influenza Preparedness: Sharing of Influenza Viruses and Access to Vaccines and Other Benefits: Report of the Advisory Group: Report by the Director-General. A65/19. Accessed 19 July 2014. http://apps.who.int/gb/ebwha/pdf_files/WHA65/A65_19-en.pdf

WHO (2012f) WHO's Response, and Role as the Health Cluster Lead, in Meeting the Growing Demands of Health in Humanitarian Emergencies: Report by the Secretariat. A65/25. Accessed 19 July 2014. http://apps.who.int/gb/ebwha/pdf_files/WHA65/A65_25-en.pdf

WHO (2012g) Address by Dr Margaret Chan, Director-General, to the Sixty-Fifth World Health Assembly. A65/3. Accessed 22 July 2014. http://apps.who.int/gb/ebwha/pdf_files/WHA65/A65_3-en.pdf

WHO (2012h) Global Mass Gatherings: Implications and Opportunities for Global Health Security: Report by the Secretariat. A65/18. Accessed 19 July 2014. http://apps.who.int/gb/ebwha/pdf_files/WHA65/A65_18-en.pdf

WHO (2013a) Implementation of the International Health Regulations (2005): Report by the Director-General. A66/16. Accessed 7 July 2014. http://apps.who.int/gb/ebwha/pdf_files/WHA66/A66_16-en.pdf

WHO (2013b) Draft Twelfth General Programme of Work. A66/6. Accessed 18 July 2014. http://apps.who.int/gb/ebwha/pdf_files/WHA66/A66_6-en.pdf

WHO (2013c) Committee A: Provisional Summary Record of the Eighth Meeting. A66/A/PSR/8. Accessed 22 July 2014. http://apps.who.int/gb/ebwha/pdf_files/WHA66-PSR/A66_A_PSR8-en.pdf (Ch. 6).

WHO (2013d) Antibiotic Resistance – A Threat to Global Health Security: Side Event at the Sixty-Sixth WHA. Accessed 22 July 2014. http://www.who.int/drugresistance/activities/wha66_side_event/en/

WHO (2013e) Novel Coronavirus Infection in the United Kingdom, 22 September 2012. Accessed 23 July 2014. http://www.who.int/csr/don/2012_09_23/en/

WHO (2013f) Novel Coronavirus Infection – Update (Middle East Respiratory Syndrome – Coronavirus), 23 May 2013. Accessed 23 July 2014. http://www.who.int/csr/don/2013_05_23_ncov/en/

WHO (2013g) Naming of the Novel Coronavirus. Accessed 23 July 2014. http://www.who.int/csr/disease/coronavirus_infections/NamingCoV_28May13.pdf?ua=1

WHO (2013h) Revised Interim Case Definition for Reporting to WHO – Middle East Respiratory Syndrome Coronavirus (MERS-CoV): Interim Case Definition as of 3 July 2013. Accessed 23 July 2014. http://www.who.int/csr/disease/coronavirus_infections/case_definition/en/

WHO (2013i) Middle East Respiratory Syndrome Coronavirus (MERS-CoV) – Update, 7 July 2013. Accessed 23 July 2014. http://www.who.int/csr/don/2013_07_07/en/

WHO (2013j) Middle East Respiratory Syndrome Coronavirus (MERS-CoV): Statement by WHO Director-General, Dr Margaret Chan, 9 July 2013. Accessed 23 July 2014. http://www.who.int/ihr/procedures/statements_20130709/en/

WHO (2013k) Committee A: Provisional Summary Record of the Seventh Meeting. A66/A/PSR/7. Accessed 23 July 2014. http://apps.who.int/gb/ebwha/pdf_files/WHA66-PSR/A66_A_PSR7-en.pdf

WHO (2014a) HIV/AIDS: About Us. Accessed 27 July 2014. http://www.who.int/hiv/aboutdept/en/

WHO (2014b) Poliomyelitis: Intensification of the Global Eradication Initiative: Report by the Secretariat. A67/38. Accessed 14 July 2014. http://apps.who.int/gb/ebwha/pdf_files/WHA67/A67_38-en.pdf

WHO (2014c) Yellow Fever. Accessed 26 July 2014. http://www.who.int/csr/don/archive/disease/yellow_fever/en/

WHO (2014d) Global Influenza Surveillance and Response System (GISRS). Accessed 13 May 2014. http://www.who.int/influenza/gisrs_laboratory/en/

WHO (2014e) Avian Influenza. Fact Sheet: Updated March 2014. Accessed 27 July 2014. http://www.who.int/mediacentre/factsheets/avian_influenza/en/

WHO (2014f) Implementation of the International Health Regulations (2005): Report by the Director-General. Accessed 7 July 2014. http://apps.who.int/gb/ebwha/pdf_files/WHA67/A67_35-en.pdf

WHO (2014g) Health has an Obligatory Place on Any Post-2015 Agenda: Dr Margaret Chan, Director-General of the World Health Organization: Address to the Sixty-Seventh World Health Assembly. Accessed 22 July 2014. http://www.who.int/dg/speeches/2014/wha-19052014/en/

WHO (2014h) Implementation of the International Health Regulations (2005): Report by the Director-General. A67/35. Accessed 23 July 2014. http://apps.who.int/gb/ebwha/pdf_files/WHA67/A67_35-en.pdf

WHO (2014i) *Antimicrobial Resistance: Global Report on Surveillance.* Geneva: World Health Organization.

WHO (2014j) WHO Statement on the Seventh Meeting of the IHR Emergency Committee Regarding MERS-CoV. Accessed 7 November 2014. http://who.int/mediacentre/news/statements/2014/7th-mers-emergency-committee/en/

WHO (2014k) Ground Zero in Guinea: The Outbreak Smoulders – Undetected – For More Than Three Months: A Retrospective on the First Cases of the Outbreak. Accessed 2 October 2014. http://www.who.int/csr/disease/ebola/ebola-6-months/guinea/en/

WHO (2014l) Ebola Virus Disease in Guinea. Accessed 2 October 2014. http://www.who.int/csr/don/2014_03_23_ebola/en/

WHO (2014m) Ebola Virus Disease in Liberia. Accessed 2 October 2014. http://www.who.int/csr/don/2014_03_30_ebola_lbr/en/

WHO (2014n) Ebola Virus Disease, West Africa – Update. Accessed 2 October 2014. http://www.who.int/csr/don/2014_04_01_ebola/en/

WHO (2014o) Statement on the 1st Meeting of the IHR Emergency Committee on the 2014 Ebola Outbreak in West Africa. Accessed 8 November 2014. http://www.who.int/mediacentre/news/statements/2014/ebola-20140808/en/

WHO (2014p) Ebola Response Roadmap Situation Report 1, 29 August 2014. Accessed 8 November 2014. http://apps.who.int/iris/bitstream/10665/131974/1/roadmapsitrep1_eng.pdf?ua=1

WHO (2014q) WHO Response to Internal Ebola Document Leaked to Media. Accessed 8 November 2014. http://www.who.int/mediacentre/news/statements/2014/ebola_document_leak/en/

WHO (2014r) UN senior leaders outline needs for global Ebola response. Accessed 8 November 2014. http://www.who.int/mediacentre/news/releases/2014/ebola-response-needs/en/

WHO AFRO (2009a) *WHO Country Cooperation Strategy: Malawi.* Brazzaville: WHO Regional Office for Africa. Accessed 18 July 2014. http://www.who.int/countryfocus/cooperation_strategy/ccs_mwi_en.pdf

WHO AFRO (2009b) *WHO Country Cooperation Strategy: Lesotho.* Brazzaville: WHO Regional Office for Africa. Accessed 18 July 2014. http://www.who.int/countryfocus/cooperation_strategy/ccs_lso_en.pdf

WHO AFRO (2009c) *WHO Country Cooperation Strategy: Swaziland.* Brazzaville: WHO Regional Office for Africa. Accessed 18 July 2014. http://www.who.int/countryfocus/cooperation_strategy/ccs_swz_en.pdf

WHO AFRO (2009d) *WHO Country Cooperation Strategy: Mauritius.* Brazzaville: WHO Regional Office for Africa. Accessed 18 July 2014. http://www.who.int/countryfocus/cooperation_strategy/ccs_mus_en.pdf

WHO AFRO (2014) Dr Matshidiso Moeti of Botswana Nominated New World Health Organization's Regional Director for Africa. Accessed 8 November 2014. http://www.afro.who.int/en/media-centre/pressreleases/item/7145-dr-matshidiso-moeti-of-botswana-nominated-new-world-health-organization%E2%80%99s-regional-director-for-africa.html

WHO Commission on Macroeconomics and Health (2001) *Macroeconomics and Health: Investing in Health for Economic Development. Report of the Commission on Macroeconomics and Health.* Geneva: World Health Organization.

WHO EB (2001) Global Health Security – Epidemic Alert and Response: Revision of the International Health Regulations. EB107/INF.DOC./7. Accessed 8 April 2014. http://apps.who.int/gb/archive/e/e_eb107.html

WHO EB (2006a) Strengthening Pandemic Influenza Preparedness and Response: Strengthening Health and Surveillance Systems: Use of Information Technology and Geographical Information Systems. EB117/32. Accessed 3 June 2014.

WHO EB (2006b) Avian and Pandemic Influenza: Developments, Response and Follow-Up, and Application of the International Health Regulations (2005): Report by the Secretariat. EB120/15. Accessed 3 June 2014. http://apps.who.int/gb/ebwha/pdf_files/EB120/b120_15-en.pdf

WHO EB (2007) Executive Board 119th Session: Geneva, 6–8 November 2006: Summary Records. 120th Session: Geneva, 22–29 January 2007: Summary Records. EB119/2206-EB120/2007/REC/2. Accessed 21 July 2014. http://apps.who.int/gb/ebwha/pdf_files/EB119-EB120-REC2/EN/B119_120_Rec2-en.pdf

WHO EB (2008a) Executive Board: 122nd Session: Geneva, 21–25 January 2008: Summary Records. EB122/2008/REC/2. Accessed 18 July 2014. http://apps.who.int/gb/ebwha/pdf_files/EB122-REC2/B122_REC_2-en.pdf

WHO EB (2008b) *Executive Board 122nd Session: Geneva, 21–25 January 2008: Resolutions and Decisions, Annexes.* Geneva: World Health Organization. Accessed 18 July 2014. http://apps.who.int/gb/ebwha/pdf_files/EB122_2008_REC1/B122_2008_REC1-en.pdf

WHO EB (2009) Executive Board: 124th Session: Geneva, 19–26 January 2009: Summary Records. EB124/2009/REC/2. Accessed 22 July 2014. http://apps.who.int/gb/ebwha/pdf_files/EB124-REC2/B124_REC2-en.pdf

WHO EB (2010a) Executive Board: 126th Session: Geneva, 18–26 January 2010: Summary Records. EB126/2010/REC/2. Accessed 22 July 2014. http://apps.who.int/gb/ebwha/pdf_files/EB126-REC2/B126_REC2-en.pdf

WHO EB (2010b) The Future Financing for WHO: Summary of a Consultation: Report by the Secretariat. EB128/INF.DOC./2. Accessed 19 July 2014. http://apps.who.int/gb/ebwha/pdf_files/EB128/B128_ID2-en.pdf

WHO EB (2010c) The Future Financing for WHO: Report by the Director-General. EB128/21. Accessed 19 July 2014. http://apps.who.int/gb/ebwha/pdf_files/EB128/B128_21-en.pdf

WHO EB (2011a) WHO Reform. EBSS/2/INF.DOC./4. Accessed 19 July 2014. http://apps.who.int/gb/ebwha/pdf_files/EBSS/EBSS2_ID4-en.pdf

WHO EB (2011b) WHO Reform. EBSS/2/INF.DOC./5. Accessed 19 July 2014. http://apps.who.int/gb/ebwha/pdf_files/EBSS/EBSS2_ID5-en.pdf

WHO EB (2011c) WHO Reform. EBSS/2/INF.DOC./6. Accessed 19 July 2014. http://apps.who.int/gb/ebwha/pdf_files/EBSS/EBSS2_ID6-en.pdf

WHO EB (2011d) Executive Board: 128th Session: Geneva, 17–24 January 2011: Summary Records. EB128/2011/REC/2. Accessed 22 July 2014. http://apps.who.int/gb/ebwha/pdf_files/EB128-REC2/B128_REC2-en.pdf

WHO EB (2011e) Programmatic Priorities: Introductory Remarks by the Director-General. EBSS/2/INF.DOC./10. Accessed 22 July 2014. http://apps.who.int/gb/ebwha/pdf_files/EBSS/EBSS2_ID10-en.pdf

WHO EB (2012) Executive Board: 130th Session: Geneva, 16–23 January 2012: Summary Records. EB130/2012/REC/2. Accessed 22 July 2014. http://apps.who.int/gb/ebwha/pdf_files/EB130-REC2/B130_2012_REC2-en.pdf

WHO EB (2013) Executive Board: 132nd Session: Geneva, 21–29 January 2013: Summary Records, List of Participants. EB132/2013/REC/2. Accessed 22 July 2014. http://apps.who.int/gb/ebwha/pdf_files/EB132-REC2/B132_REC2-en.pdf

Williams MC (2003) Words, Images, Enemies: Securitization and International Politics. *International Studies Quarterly*, 47(4): 511–31.

World Bank (2014) Transcript of Remarks at the Event: Impact of the Ebola Crisis: A Perspective from the Countries. The World Bank. Accessed 10 November 2014. http://www.worldbank.org/en/news/speech/2014/10/09/transcript-event-impact-ebola-crisis-perspective-countries

WTO (2011) Committee on Sanitary and Phytosanitary Measures – Specific Trade Concerns – Note by the Secretariat – Issues Not Considered in 2010 – Addendum. G/SPS/GEN/204/Rev.11/Add.2. Accessed 6 May 2014. http://docsonline.wto.org/gen_home.asp

Yamey G (2002a) Head of WHO to Stand Down. *BMJ*, 325(7362): 457.

Yamey G (2002b) WHO in 2002: Have the Latest Reforms Reversed WHO's Decline? *BMJ*, 325(7372): 1107–12.

Yamey G (2002c) WHO in 2002: Interview with Gro Harlem Brundtland. *BMJ*, 325(7376): 1356.

Yamey G and Abbasi K (2003) New Leader, New Hope for WHO. *BMJ*, 326(7399): 1100.

Yekutiel P (1981) Lessons from the Big Eradication Campaigns. *World Health Forum*, 2(4): 465–90.

Youde J (2012) *Global Health Governance*. Cambridge: Polity.

Index

Page numbers in **bold** refer to Table 6.1.

agency slack, 182, 186, 190
   adoption of security discourse by
      WHO, 11
   institutional design, 10
   management of SARS outbreak by
      WHO, 22, 154
   organizational autonomy, 10
   preference heterogeneity, 10
   principal-agent theory, 9–10
   shirking, and WHO, 10, 14:
      avoidance of directing-
      authority role, 74, 77;
      influenza programme, 129, 132,
      138, 148; Smallpox Eradication
      Programme, 56; suppression of
      security discourse, 168, 179, 185
   slippage, and WHO, 9–10, 14:
      adoption of security discourse, 86;
      focus on infectious diseases, 31;
      management of Ebola outbreak,
      178; suppression of security
      discourse, 164, 182
Amsterdam Conference (2000), 70
Annan, Kofi, 136
antimicrobial resistance (AMR), 164,
   169–70, 190
Asian Flu pandemic (1957), 127–8
Association of South East Asian
   Nations (ASEAN), 138
Aum Shinrikyo terrorist attack, 107

Bacille Calmette-Guérin (BCG)
   vaccine, 66
Balzacq, T, 13–14
Banbury, Anthony, 177
Barnett, M, 37
Beales, P, 49
Beigbeder, Y, 39, 94
Bekedam, Henk, 97
belief structures, influence on global
   health policy, 8–9, 16

Biological and Toxic Weapons
   Convention (BWC), 116
biological weapons, 106–7
bird flu, *see* H5N1 avian influenza
Bøås, M, 13
Brazil, 5, 158, 159, 167
Brés, P, 104
Brundtland, Gro Harlem, 80–1, 97, 98,
   111, 117, 136, 174
Burci, GL, 40, 91
Buzan, B, 12, 13, 182–3, 185

Calder, R, 27
Candau, Marcolino, 56
capacity gaps, and global health,
   188–9
Carter, I, 105
Cassels, Andrew, 139
Cavaillon, Andre, 65–6
Central Intelligency Agency (CIA),
   41–2
Centres for Disease Control and
   Prevention (CDC) (United States),
   58, 93, 140
Chan, Margaret, 130–1, 139, 141–4,
   168–70, 173, 177
chemical, biological, radiological or
   nuclear (CBRN) events, 121
chemical weapons, 106–7
China, SARS outbreak, 87, 89–90, 96
   WHO's criticism of, 97–8, 173–4
Chisholm, Brock, 55
cholera, 106
Chung-Li, Hu, 109–10
civil rights, and health, 23–4, 26
Cocksedge, Sandy, 113, 114, 147
Commission on Macroeconomics and
   Health, 42
Committee on International
   Epidemiology and Quarantine,
   102

Communicable Disease
    Surveillance and Response
    Unit (CSR), 81–2
  outbreak verification strategy, 82–4,
    112–14
  use of non-governmental
    information, 82–4, 113–14
constructivism, 9, 14, 186
Copenhagen School, and
    securitization theory,
    12–14, 182–3
Cordingley, Peter, 97
customary international law, 30,
    117–18

Davies, S, 155–6
DDT, and malaria control and
    eradication, 46, 47, 50–1
delegation contract, and WHO's
    disease eradication mandate, 21,
    28, 30, 43, 78, 101
  desecuritization of, 185
  revision of, 79, 82, 84–6, 99, 108,
    149, 170
Delon, PJ, 105
dengue haemorrhagic fever, 104
desecuritization, 183
  categories of, 183
  Huysmans dilemma, 184
  problems with, 184–5
Directly Observed Treatment,
    Short-course (DOTS), 69, 71
director-general of the WHO, 16
  emergency powers, 33
  issuing of recommendation, 120
disease surveillance, 169
  epidemic intelligence, 89
  importance of timely data, 88–9
  intelligence coordination, 88–91
  problems with, 88
  see also Communicable Disease
    Surveillance and Response Unit;
    Global Influenza Surveillance
    Network; Global Outbreak Alert
    and Response Network
distal principals, and WHO, 11,
    115, 135, 176

Ebola Virus Disease (EVD), in West
    Africa, 104, 106, 174–9, 185

criticism of WHO's response,
    176–8
  military intervention, 175, 189
  United Nations response, 175–7
  WHO's response to, 175–7
Egypt, 141, 146
Elbe, S, 6
Emerging and Other Communicable
    Diseases (EMC) unit, 81, 108–9
  see also Communicable
    Disease Surveillance and
    Response Unit
Enemark, C, 6
epistemic communities, 82, 111, 147
  global community of health
    professionals, 157
  organizational learning, 45, 86
  Smallpox Eradication Programme, 58
  tuberculosis control programmes, 72
European Commission, 138
  Health Security Committee, 3
Executive Board (EB) (of WHO), 16
  authority to grant emergency
    powers to director-general, 33
  criticism of securitization of
    health, 159–60
Expert Committee on Influenza, 126,
    127
Expert Committee on International
    Quarantine, 103
Expert Committee on Respiratory
    Virus Diseases, 128

Fenner, F, 60
Fidler, DP, 100
Fineberg, Harvey, 144
Finnemore, M, 37
Fischer, F, 13
FluNet, 131
Food and Agriculture Organization
    (FAO), 135, 137
frames/framing, 12–13
  desecuritization, 183
  new concept of security, 84
  reframing influenza as security
    threat, 138
  reframing of WHO's public health
    mandate, 85, 123, 151, 158, 164,
    168, 179, 181, 183–5
  relationship with public policy, 13

France, 158
Fukuda, Keiji, 142, 173
functionalism, and post-war
    world-view, 22–3

G8, 18
G20, 18
Gagnon, M, 157
geographical information system
    (GIS), 83
Giesecke, Johan, 113
Gilles, H, 49
Global Agenda on Influenza
    Surveillance and Control (2002),
    131–2
Global DOTS Expansion Plan (GDEP),
    71
global financial crisis (2008), impact
    on WHO, 162
Global Fund for HIV/AIDS,
    Tuberculosis and Malaria, 18, 75
global health governance (GHG), 9
global health security
    change in approach to disease
        outbreaks, 4, 79
    consensus over core features of,
        14–15
    critiques of concept, 4–6, 20, 151,
        152, 178–9, 182: academic
        community, 5–6, 152–8; criticism
        of WHO, 155–6; Executive Board
        of WHO, 159–60; limited
        criticism of WHO, 154–5; member
        states, 4–5, 158–63, 182; reasons
        for limited criticism, 156–8;
        security sector, 6, 154; social
        justice, 153; Western dominance,
        152–3
    definition of, 3, 15, 85, 188:
        resolving problems with,
        187–8
    expanded scope of concept, 3–4
    origins of concept, 2–3, 24–5,
        84–5
    widespread adoption of concept, 3,
        151, 153, 154, 157–8, 166, 167
    see also securitization of health,
        and WHO
Global Health Security Agenda, 3
Global Health Security Initiative, 3

Global Influenza Surveillance
    and Response System (GISRS),
    127
Global Influenza Surveillance Network
    (GISN), 89, 126–7, 133
globalization, impact of, 2, 187
Global Outbreak Alert and Response
    Network (GOARN), 84, 89,
    114–15, 133
    revision of International Health
    Regulations, 115–16
    support for, 86
Global Polio Eradication Initiative
    (GPEI), 41–2
Global Public Health Information
    Network (GPHIN), 83, 89, 112
Global TB Drug Facility (GDF), 73
Godlee, Fiona, 107, 157
Graham, ER, 11, 14
Guinea, 174
Gutteridge, Frank, 103

H1N1 influenza pandemic (2009), 20,
    125, 126, 140–8
    controversy over WHO's role, 22
    IHR Emergency Committee, 141,
        142
    origins of, 140–1
    unilateral trade and travel
        restrictions, 141, 145
    WHO's response to, 141–3, 170–1:
        accusations of improper conduct,
        144; announcement of pandemic,
        142; avoids criticism of member
        states, 145–8, 171; avoids
        prescriptive approach, 143;
        coordinating role, 143–4;
        criticism of, 141–2, 144–5; failure
        to enforce IHR compliance,
        145–8, 171; as lead technical
        agency, 143
H5N1 avian influenza, 20, 125, 126
    Hong Kong outbreak (1997), 125–6,
        130–1
    impact on WHO's influenza
        programme, 130–1, 133
    Indonesia, 158–9
    member states' lack of preparedness,
        135
    securitization of, 136–9

H5N1 avian influenza – *continued*
　WHO's response to reappearance of,
　　133–4, 138: avoids criticism of
　　member states, 134–6;
　　coordinating role, 137, 138;
　　Influenza Pandemic Task Force,
　　137, 138; Inter-Governmental
　　Meeting, 136–8
H7N9 avian influenza, 133
H8 (Health 8), 18
Haas, EB, 45, 86
Hanrieder, T, 156
Hansen, L, 183, 184
Hardiman, Max, 115
Health Canada, 83
HealthMapper, 83
health, WHO's definition of, 27,
　31, 43
　health security, 164
Henderson, Donald, 58, 60, 62, 64, 65
Heymann, David, 82, 86, 96, 106,
　136, 147
　revision of International Health
　　Regulations, 108–10
HIV/AIDS, 6, 17–19, 29–30, 67, 69,
　104
Hoffman, SJ, 187
Hogan, R, 128
Hong Kong Flu pandemic (1968), 128
human security, criticism of
　concept, 6
Huysmans, Jeff, 184
Hwenda, L, 187

ideas, influence on health policy, 8–9,
　16
India, 159
Indonesia, 5, 146–7, 158–9, 167
influenza, and WHO, 125–6, 148–9
　approach during 1950s, 126–30:
　　agency shirking, 129, 132, 138,
　　148; classical approach to
　　infectious diseases, 128–30;
　　declining interest in, 128–9;
　　Global Influenza Surveillance
　　Network, 126–7; intelligence
　　coordination, 129–30; policy
　　advice, 130; public health focus
　　of, 130; vaccination, 127–8

factors explaining lack of urgency
　over, 132
fluctuation of political interest in,
　131
Global Agenda on Influenza
　Surveillance and Control, 131–2
Guidelines on Vaccine and Antiviral
　Use during Influenza Pandemics,
　132
intelligence coordination, 134
member states' lack of preparedness,
　135
pandemic potential, 133
real-time policy advice, 134
reframing as security threat, 138
securitization of, 125, 126, 136–9,
　149
United Nations System Influenza
　Coordinator, 135–6
see also H1N1 influenza pandemic
　(2009); H5N1 avian influenza
Influenza Pandemic Task Force, 137,
　138
institutional design
　agency slack, 10
　international organizations, 10
　World Health Organization, 15–16,
　　35, 36
intellectual property, 173
intelligence coordination
　disease surveillance, 88, 169:
　　importance of timely data, 88–9
　epidemic intelligence, 89
　Global Influenza Surveillance
　　Network, 126–7
　H5N1 avian influenza, 134
　International Health Regulations, 122
　SARS outbreak, 89–91: virtual global
　　networks, 90–1
Inter-Governmental Meeting (2005),
　and H5N1 influenza virus, 137, 138
Intergovernmental Working Group
　(IGWG), revision of International
　Health Regulations, 117–22
Interim Commission of the World
　Health Organization, 27, 29,
　31–2, 102
　Expert Committee on Malaria, 46–8
　tuberculosis, 65–6

International Atomic Energy Agency
(IAEA), 121
International Civil Aviation
Organization (ICAO), 35–6
International Health Conference
(1946), 31, 34
International Health Regulations
Emergency Committee,
119–21, 170
accusations of political
interference, 121
Ebola outbreak in West Africa, 175
H1N1 influenza pandemic, 141,
142: accusations of improper
conduct, 144
Middle East Respiratory Syndrome,
172
International Health Regulations
(IHR), 3, 20, 29, 81, 126
adoption of revised framework
(2005), 122–3
changes to list of notifiable
diseases, 104
concern over WHO's real-time
principal policy adviser role,
118–19
concerns over state sovereignty,
117, 134–5, 170
failure to enforce in H1N1
pandemic, 145–8, 171
global health security, 123
importance of, 101
influenza monitoring, 126
lack of interest in amending, 104–5
member states' non-compliance, 105
origins of, 102–4
Public Health Emergency of
International Concern, 113,
118–20
real-time intelligence
coordination, 122, 169
revision of, 101–2, 121: beginning
of process, 109–16; delays, 110,
115, 116; factors encouraging,
106–8; impact of Brundtland's
appointment, 111–12; informal
consultation group, 109–10;
Intergovernmental Working
Group negotiations, 117–22;

member states' lack of
enthusiasm, 110–11; merging
with GOARN team, 115–16;
renewed support for, 116–17
scope and terms of, 103, 104
securitization of health, 101–2, 123
voluntary compliance with, 137
WHO's role as government assessor
and critic, 120–2
International Monetary Fund (IMF), 18
international organizations (IOs)
authority of, 4–6, 15
autonomy of, 10
as complex entities, 11
constraints on, 10
criticisms of, 6–7
customary international law, 30,
117–18
delegation contract, 21
distal principals, 11
functional approach to world order,
22–3
influence of people's ideas and
beliefs, 16
institutional design, 10
'mission creep', 4
principal-agent relationships, 10–11
principal-agent theory, 9–10
proximal principals, 11
studies of, 7
International Relations (IR)
agency/structure debate, 17
study of international
organizations, 7
International Sanitary Bureau, 27
International Sanitary Conference, 25,
33, 103
International Sanitary Regulations
(ISR), 29
origins and adoption of, 102–3
problems with, 103
renamed International Health
Regulations, 103–4
revision of, 103–4
scope and terms of, 103
see also International Health
Regulations
International Society for Infectious
Diseases, 83

Jensen, K, 128
Jin, J, 155
Johnson, Lyndon B, 58

Karackattu, JT, 155
Kreuder-Sonnen, C, 156

Labonté, R, 157
League of Nations, 26
League of Nations Health
    Organization (LNHO), 26, 27, 126
League of Red Cross Societies, 25
Lee, Jong-wook, 136
Legionnaires' disease, 104
Leong, Hoe Nam, 1–2, 90, 92
Liberia, 174
Lyne, MM, 10

Maclean, S, 5, 6
McNeill, D, 13
Mahler, Haflan, 65
Malaria Eradication Programme
    (MEP), 19, 45–54
  achievements of, 49
  closure of, 49
  command-and-control approach,
    48–9
  DDT residual spraying, 50–2
  donor disillusionment, 50
  exclusion of malaria-endemic
    regions, 52
  Expert Committee on Malaria, 46–8
  failure of, 46, 49, 54: lessons learned
    from, 59–61, 78
  financing of, 46
  governance style of WHO:
    government assessor, 54;
    intelligence consolidator, 53;
    policy prescriber, 53–4
  impact on WHO's reputation, 53–4
  inflexibility of strategy, 51–2
  insecticide resistance, 51
  launch of, 46
  limitations of, 50–2
  malaria control policy, 47:
    eradication, 47–8
  methodology, 48
  origins of, 46–7
  procedural protocols, 48

Mann, Jonathan, 107
material transfer agreements, 173
Médecins Sans Frontières (MSF), 174–5
Memish, ZA, 173
Mexico, H1N1 influenza pandemic
    (2009), 140–1
Middle East Respiratory Syndrome
    (MERS-CoV), 171–2
  WHO's management of, 172–4
  military intervention, 189
  Ebola outbreak in West Africa, 175,
    189
Millennium Development Goals
    (MDGs), 42–3, 131
'mission creep', 4, 10, 38
Mitrany, David, 22–3
Moran, M, 154

Nabarro, David, 136
Nakajima, Hiroshi, 69, 107–9, 111
National Influenza Centres (NICs),
    126–7
Nelson, TE, 12–13
neo-colonialism, and securitization of
    health, 152–3
Nigeria, 41, 174, 175
non-governmental information, and
    outbreak verification strategy,
    82–4, 113–14
Norway, 158
notifiable diseases, 29, 103, 104

Obama, Barack, 175
Oestreich, J, 14, 16, 185–6
Office Internationale d'Hygiene
    Publique (OIHP), 25–7, 126
official development assistance (ODA),
    growth in, 166
organizational learning
  epistemic communities, 45, 86
  Smallpox Eradication Programme,
    59–60
Oslo Declaration (2007), 158
Oswald, SU, 154–5
outbreak verification strategy, 82–4,
    112–14
  use of non-governmental
    information, 82–4, 113–14
Oxley, ZM, 12–13

Pakistan, 41–2
Pan American Health Organization
  (PAHO), 26
Pan American Sanitary Bureau
  (PASB), 27, 47, 55
Pan American Sanitary Conferences,
  27, 29
Pan American Sanitary Organization
  (PASO), 26, 27
Pan Arab Regional Health Bureau, 26
Pandemic Influenza Preparedness
  (PIP) Framework, 3, 127
plague, 106
post-structuralism, 14, 152–3
poverty reduction, 42–3
preference heterogeneity, 10, 11, 14,
  182, 186, 187
Primary Health Care movement, 105
principal-agent theory, 9–11, 186
  relationship in international
    organizations, 10–11
  securitization theory, 14
  see also agency slack; distal
    principals; proximal principals
Pro-MED, 83
proximal principals, and WHO, 11,
  58, 86–7, 115, 135, 146, 151, 152,
  176, 178, 190
Public Health Emergency of
  International Concern (PHEIC),
  113, 118–20, 175, 188

Qatar, 171
quarantine, 25, 103

Raska, Karel, 57–8, 60
rationalist approaches, 14, 186
Rein, M, 12
relapsing fever, 104
Rockefeller Foundation, 47
Rodier, Guénaël, 85, 96, 106, 111,
  113, 115–17, 147
Ryan, Mike, 111–12, 114, 147

SARS (Severe Acute Respiratory
  Syndrome), 2003 outbreak,
  1–2, 20, 87–8
  global economic impact, 79
  mortality, 79

securitization of, 20, 79
  successful containment of, 91, 99
  WHO's handling of: advice to
    individual travellers, 93, 95, 96,
    118; classical approach, 88;
    control of human-to-human
    transmission, 93; controversy
    over, 22, 93; criticism of China,
    97–8, 173–4; as government
    assessor/critic, 94–9; real-time
    intelligence coordination, 88–91;
    real-time principal policy adviser,
    91–3; screening of travellers,
    92–3; significance of, 99–100;
    Taiwan, 98–9; virtual global
    networks, 90–1
Schön, DA, 12
secretariat of World Health
  Organization, 16
  autonomy of, 36–8: concerns over,
    117, 134–5
  classical approach to disease
    eradication, 45–6
  disease eradication obligation,
    28, 43
  as government assessor/critic,
    120–2
  issuing of recommendation, 120
  real-time intelligence coordination,
    122
  reputational power and authority,
    41
  revision of International Health
    Regulations, 108, 116, 120
  see also World Health Organization
securitization of health, and WHO,
  2–3, 85–6, 151–2
  benefits of, 165, 181, 184, 187:
    financial and political support,
    165–6; growth in official
    development assistance, 166;
    recognition of health as foreign
    policy issue, 165
  concerns over, 5–6
  criticisms of, 4, 20, 151, 152, 178–9,
    182: academic community, 5–6,
    152–8; criticism of WHO, 155–6;
    impact on General Programme of
    Work, 160, **161**–2; Indonesia and

securitization of health – *continued*
   H5N1 virus-sharing, 158–9;
   involvement of security
   personnel, 153; limited criticism
   of WHO, 154–5; member states,
   4–5, 158–63, 182; reasons for
   limited criticism, 156–8; reform of
   objectives, 162–4; security sector,
   6, 154; social justice, 153; Western
   dominance, 152–3; within WHO's
   Executive Board, 159–60
definition of global health security,
   3, 15, 85, 188: resolving problems
   with, 187–8
influenza, 125, 126, 136–9, 149
International Health Regulations,
   101–2, 123
member states' attitudes towards:
   criticisms of, 158–63;
   inconsistency, 167; support for, 167
resolving definitional problems,
   187–8
SARS outbreak, 20, 79
suppression of health-as-security
   discourse, 162–4, 168, 182:
   desecuritization by rearticulation,
   183–4; omission of 'health
   security' in programme of work,
   160, **161**–2; possible consequences
   of, 168, 179; problems with
   desecuritization, 184–5
WHA Resolution WHA54.14 *Global
   Health Security*, 84–7
securitization theory, 12
breakdown of public policy
   processes, 182–3
components of, 12, 13
context, 13–14
desecuritization, 183: categories
   of, 183; Huysmans dilemma, 184
frames, 12–13
hyper-politicization, 183
principal-agent theory, 14
Selgelid, M, 6
Senegal, 158, 174
Shanghai, 96
Sharp, WR, 38, 40
Sierra Leone, 174
slack, *see* agency slack

Smallpox Eradication Programme
   (SEP), 19, 45, 54–65
absence of government assessment
   role, 64
accounting practices, 63
detached leadership by WHO, 56–7:
   pressures to change, 57–8; reasons
   for, 57
detection of new cases, 62
disease surveillance, 61–2
epistemic community, 58
flexible approach, 60, 62
governance style of WHO, 59–64
initial rejection of, 55
initial strategy, 56
intelligence coordination, 63–4
Intensified Smallpox Eradication
   Programme, 59
lack of interest in, 55, 74
lessons learned from failures of
   other programmes, 59–61
local autonomy, 61, 63
origins of, 55–6
policy advisory role of WHO, 61, 63
prevention of re-allocation of
   regional funds, 62–3
reporting and surveillance system,
   60–1
research into new methods of
   eradication, 61
response to epidemics, 62
Smallpox Eradication Unit, 57–60
strategy of, 59
success of, 54–5, 64–5
technical assistance, 60
transformation in management of,
   58–9
social justice, and criticism of
   securitization of health, 153
social medicine, and origins of World
   Health Organization, 23–4, 26–7
social welfare
link with international security, 24
origins of World Health
   Organization, 24, 26
Soper, Fred, 55
South Africa, 158
Spanish influenza pandemic (1918),
   126, 130

Special Committee on International
    Sanitary Regulations, 102
Sri Lanka, 167
Stephenson, N, 154
Stevenson, M, 154
Stop TB Partnership, 70–3
    Amsterdam Conference (2000), 70
    governance style, 71–3
    WHO's relationship with, 72–3
    WHO's role, 71, 72, 75
Surat (India), 106
swine flu, *see* H1N1 influenza
    pandemic (2009)
syndromic reporting system, 110, 111

Taiwan, 98–9
Taliban, 41–2
terrorism, 107
Thailand, 5, 158–60, 167
tuberculosis (TB), 19, 29
    Amsterdam Conference (2000), 70
    combination therapies, 66
    declaration of global emergency by
        WHO (1994), 69
    decline in WHO's capacity to deal
        with, 67–8
    declining interest by developed
        world, 67–9
    in developing world, 66
    Directly Observed Treatment,
        Short-course, 69, 71
    director-general's report on global
        situation (1993), 68–9
    epistemic community, 72
    Expert Committee on Tuberculosis,
        66, 67
    Global DOTS Expansion Plan, 71
    Global TB Drug Facility, 73
    intelligence role of WHO, 72
    multi-drug-resistant-tuberculosis,
        67
    postwar vaccination campaign, 66
    resurgence of, 67–8
    WHO's neglect of, 65
    WHO's postwar concern over, 65–6
    World Health Assembly strategy
        (1991), 68
    see also Stop TB Partnership
typhus, 104

UNAIDS (Joint United Nations
    Programme on HIV/AIDS), 18, 69,
    107, 135–6
Union of Soviet Socialist Republics
    (USSR), and Smallpox Eradication
    Programme, 55–6
United Kingdom, 152, 157
United Nations, and specialized
    agencies, 35–6
United Nations Children's Emergency
    Fund (UNICEF), 47, 50, 66, 83, 135
United Nations Development
    Programme (UNDP), 84, 135
United Nations Educational, Scientific
    and Cultural Organization
    (UNESCO), 23
United Nations Mission for Ebola
    Emergency Response (UNMEER),
    175–7
United Nations Relief and
    Rehabilitation Administration
    (UNRRA), 26, 27, 47
United Nations Security Council, 121
    Ebola outbreak, 175–6
United Nations System Influenza
    Coordinator (UNSIC), 135–6, 143
United States, 58, 68, 151, 152
Urbani, Carlo, 90, 97

vector control programmes, 51, 57
Velimirovic, B, 103
Venice, 25
Vietnam, 95
Vignes, C, 40, 91

weaver, V, 10
Weir, L, 84, 85
Whelan, Mary, 117–19
World Bank, 18, 135, 137
    autonomy of, 35
World Health Assembly (WHA), 16,
    17, 29
    authority of, 39
    delegates, 36
    exceptional regulatory powers of,
        32–3
    health security, definition of, 164
    information-gathering and
        categorization, 32

World Health Assembly – *continued*
  regulations of, 32
  resolutions of, 30
  resolution WHA4.75 *International Sanitary Regulations*, 29
  resolution WHA8.30 *Malaria Eradication*, 46
  resolution WHA48.7 *Revision of the International Health Regulations*, 81–2, 108
  resolution WHA48.13 *Communicable Disease Prevention and Control*, 82, 84, 85, 108
  resolution WHA54.14 *Global Health Security*, 84, 85, 87, 114, 122
  resolution WHA56.28 *Revision of the International Health Regulations*, 116
  resolution WHA58.3 *Revision of the International Health Regulations*, 101, 123
  resolution WHA59.2 *Application of the International Health Regulations*, 137–8
  Smallpox Eradication Programme, 55–6
  tuberculosis, 68
World Health Organization (WHO)
  advisory function of, 15, 75–6, 91–2: concerns over role, 118–19; Malaria Eradication Programme, 53–4; SARS outbreak, 92–3; Smallpox Eradication Programme, 61, 63
  authority of: constraints on, 15, 38–43, 78, 94; delegated authority, 21, 34; directing and coordinating, 2, 4, 21, 34–5, 43, 53, 78, 169; reluctance to act as directing authority, 74, 78, 138; types of, 15
  autonomy of, 33, 35, 37–8: concerns over, 117, 134–5; constraints on, 38–43, 174; secretariat, 36–8
  Brundtland's reforms, 81
  classical approach to disease eradication, 45, 73–8, 129–30, 181
  collaborative partnerships, 91
  constraints on, 38, 43, 77, 78, 80, 170, 174, 179, 182, 189–90: budget, 40; economic, 39–40; member states' sovereignty, 38–9; polio eradication initiative, 41–2; politico-legal, 38–9; poverty reduction, 42–3; World Health Assembly, 39
  crisis of confidence in, 69–70, 80, 107–8
  delegation contract, 30, 78, 101: desecuritization of, 185; revision of, 79, 82, 84–6, 99, 108, 149, 170
  disease eradication mandate, 7–8, 43, 181: central importance of, 21, 32–3; customary international law, 30, 117–18; directing and coordinating role, 34–5; emergency powers, 33; explanation of focus on, 30–4; extension beyond notifiable diseases, 29–30; fluidity of, 28, 30, 101; historical development of, 29; International Sanitary/Health Regulations, 29; member states' interests, 34; WHA resolutions, 30
  distal principals, 11, 115, 135, 176
  epidemic intelligence consolidator role, 53, 75, 127, 128, 148
  epidemic intelligence coordinator role: disease surveillance, 88–9, 169; epidemic intelligence, 89; Global Influenza Surveillance Network, 126–7; H5N1 avian influenza, 134; International Health Regulations, 122; SARS outbreak, 89–91
  General Programme of Work, 160, **161–2**: reform of objectives, 162–4
  as government assessor/critic: avoidance of role, 64, 76, 94–5; International Health Regulations, 120–2; Malaria Eradication Programme, 54; SARS outbreak, 94–9
  health definition, 27, 31, 43: health security, 164

World Health Organization – *continued*
  historical origins, 22–8:
    dissatisfaction with existing
    institutions, 25–6; health as a civil
    right, 23–4, 26; link between
    health and security, 24–5; Mitrany
    and functionalism, 22–3; regional
    offices, 27–8; rise of social
    medicine, 23–4, 26–7
  influence of individual leaders,
    16–17, 185–6
  institutional design, 15–16, 35, 36
  as intergovernmental organization,
    34, 38
  as 'medical mafia', 37, 156–7
  member states' role, 17, 34
  'mission creep', 4–5
  objectives, reform of (2011), 162–4
  primary mission of, 15, 77–8, 181
  principal-agent theory, 10–12
  principal policy adviser role, 88,
    91–2: challenges to, 118–20; SARS
    outbreak, 92–3, 118
  proximal principals, 11, 58, 86–7,
    115, 135, 146, 151, 152, 176, 178,
    190
  regional offices, 27–8, 36
  role of, 2, 186
  A Safer Future (World Health
    Report, 2007), 3, 123, 125, 139,
    158, 159
  see also director-general of the
    WHO; Executive Board (EB);
    secretariat of World Health
    Organization; securitization of
    health, and WHO; World Health
    Assembly
World Influenza Centre (WIC),
  126
World Organization for Animal Health
  (OIE), 135, 137
World Trade Organization (WTO),
  114

Zaire, 106
Zhdanov, Viktor, 56

CPSIA information can be obtained
at www.ICGtesting.com
Printed in the USA
LVHW081933271218
601925LV00009B/96/P